Essentials of Telebehavioral Health

Hossam Mahmoud
Hady Naal • Emile Whaibeh
Editors

Essentials of Telebehavioral Health

A Practical Guide

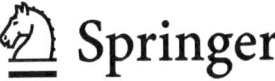 Springer

Editors
Hossam Mahmoud
Psychiatry
Tufts University School of
Medicine
Boston, MA, USA

Hady Naal
Clinical Psychology
Global Health Institute at the
American University of Beirut
Beirut, Lebanon

Emile Whaibeh
Public Health
University of Balamand
Beirut, Lebanon

ISBN 978-3-030-97324-7   ISBN 978-3-030-97325-4   (eBook)
https://doi.org/10.1007/978-3-030-97325-4

This Springer imprint is published by the registered company Springer Nature
Switzerland AG
The registered company address is: Gewerbestrasse 11, 6330 Cham, Switzerland

Contents

Editors and Contributors

About the Editors

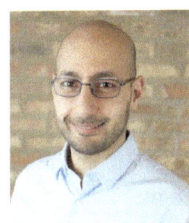

Hossam Mahmoud is a Board-Certified psychiatrist and serves as the Behavioral Health Medical Director at Cambia Health Solutions. Prior to joining Cambia, Dr. Mahmoud was the medical director and senior vice president at Array Behavioral Care (formerly InSight + Regroup), where he oversaw the planning, implementation, monitoring, and evaluation of multiple telebehavioral health programs across multiple states and a variety of clinical settings. Dr. Mahmoud is Past President of the Illinois Psychiatric Society and Distinguished Fellow of the American Psychiatric Association. He earned his Medical Degree and Master of Public Health at the American University of Beirut. He worked as a Medical Officer at the World Health Organization, before completing his residency training at McGaw Medical Center of Northwestern University in Chicago. Dr. Mahmoud has practiced psychiatry in both the United States and Canada. He holds an academic appointment at Tufts University School of Medicine. Dr. Mahmoud has worked in inpatient, outpatient, and consultation/liaison psychiatry and has been delivering telebehavioral health services since 2016. He has practiced medicine in English, French, and Arabic. In addition to telebehavioral health, Dr. Mahmoud is interested in refugee and immigrant mental health, LGBTQ mental health, and the mental health of linguistic and cultural minorities.

Tufts University School of Medicine, Boston, MA, USA

Array Behavioral Care, Mount Laurel, NJ, USA

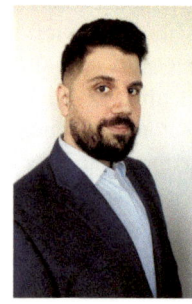

Emile Whaibeh is a Public Health Researcher based in Beirut, Lebanon. He is currently an instructor in the Department of Public Health at the University of Balamand (UOB) in the process of completing his Ph.D. degree at the Doctoral School of Science and Health [École Doctorale de Science et Santé] (EDSS) at Saint-Joseph University (USJ). His doctoral dissertation, conducted under the co-direction of both USJ and UOB is a prospective birth cohort study focused the effects of environmental exposures on birth outcomes and the physical and cognitive development of Lebanese infants. Previously, he was the lead field researcher at the Collective for Research and Training on Development-Action (CRTD.A), a Lebanese organization focused on capacity building and development projects in the Middle East and North Africa region. Additionally, he has worked on several consultancies with the private and public sectors, covering issues related to environmental health, mental health, and social determinants of health. Emile holds a master's degree in Public Health with a special focus on community health. His research interests include public mental health, environmental health, and digital health.

Department of Public Health, Faculty of Health Sciences, University of Balamand, Beirut, Lebanon

Doctoral School of Science and Health, Saint-Joseph University, Beirut, Lebanon

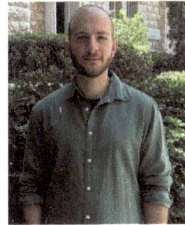

Hady Naal is a Research Consultant at the Global Health Institute at the American University of Beirut, and is an instructor at the Department of Public Health at the University of Balamand in Lebanon. He holds a Bachelor's degree in Psychology from the Lebanese American University, and a Masters' degree in Clinical Psychology from Haigazian University, where he also completed his clinical training in psychotherapy. In addition to his clinical experience, Hady has managed numerous research and public health projects for local and international non-governmental humanitarian organizations and academic institutions in Lebanon. His work has yielded multiple articles published in peer-reviewed journals focusing primarily on mental health, telebehavioral health, program evaluation, healthcare services, and health equity among others.

Global Health Institute at the American University of Beirut, Beirut, Lebanon

Contributors

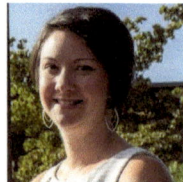

Fayth Dickenson is a Board-Certified Psychiatric Nurse who is currently a Behavioral Health Manager at Beacon Health Options. In her role, she oversees clinical quality, regulatory compliance, and business operations of a behavioral health utilization management team. Prior to her work with Beacon, she worked with other health plans and managed an inpatient adult psychiatric unit in North Central Idaho. Born and raised in the Pacific Northwest, Dickenson received her degree in nursing in 2008 and completed her Master of Healthcare Administration with Leadership Focus at Capella University in 2017. Her clinical interests include the use of telehealth to expand access to rural and under-resourced communities, suicide prevention education, and mental health stigma reduction through community education and awareness. Dickenson is a founding member and current chair of Suicide Prevention of the Inland Northwest, a grass-roots non-profit organization established to increase awareness of, educate on, and reduce stigma surrounding suicide deaths in Idaho. She has also been a certified Mental Health First Aid instructor since 2013 and has certified more than 500 individuals in adult and youth Mental Health First Aid. She currently lives in North Central Idaho with her husband and two sons where they enjoy volunteering in the community, exploring the outdoors, and traveling.

Beacon Health Options, Boston, MA, USA

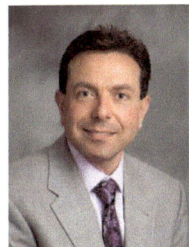

Omar Elhaj serves as Regional Medical Director at Telecare, overseeing forty programs serving underserved population in all settings of care. Prior to that, he served as Senior Medical Director at LifeStance Health where he led psychiatric clinicians providing in-person and telehealth care in 16 states. Dr. Elhaj has had extensive experience in clinical and executive leadership positions spanning different settings of health care. Dr. Elhaj is certified by the American Board of Psychiatry and Neurology in both adult psychiatry and addiction psychiatry. He earned his medical degree from Damascus University and completed his residency in general adult psychiatry at the University of Missouri at Kansas City School of Medicine, where he served as chief resident. He completed fellowships in addiction psychiatry and geriatric psychiatry at Case Western Reserve University School of Medicine, where he also served as senior research fellow in therapeutics of bipolar mood disorders. Dr. Elhaj has served as co-principal investigator for several National Institute of Mental Health (NIMH) and industry-sponsored bipolar disorder studies and has presented throughout the country on various mental health issues. He has published more than 30 peer-reviewed articles and book chapters. He currently holds the position of clinical assistant professor in the Department of Psychiatry at Case Western Reserve University School of Medicine and continues to be involved in teaching residents and fellows. He is a member of the American Medical Association and the American Psychiatric Association.

Telecare Corporation, Alamdea, CA, USA

Case Western Reserve University, Cleveland, OH, USA

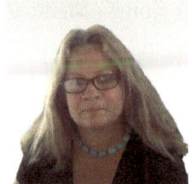

Marlene McDermott is a License Marriage and Family Therapist and the Vice-President of Therapy and Quality at Array Behavioral Care (formerly InSight + Regroup). She has over two decades of experience working in the behavioral health field and most recently, has led the direct-to-consumer telehealth practice to exponential growth. She has a vast array of clinical interests; however, her specializations include anger management, addiction, marriage and family counseling, play therapy, and stress management. Marlene was born and raised in New Jersey. She graduated from Saint Joseph's University in Philadelphia with a degree in Psychology. Marlene received her Master of Science degree from California State University, East Bay, in Educational Psychology with a focus on Marriage and Family Therapy. She has worked and managed various levels of service including home- and school-based service, residential treatment, inpatient and outpatient treatment, and was also in private practice. Marlene is currently completing a doctoral program in Developmental Psychology at Capella University. She is focused on studying an adolescent's belief in the importance of sleep and their ability to remove electronics before sleep and their relationship to sleep quality. She is also working with her passion of helping clinicians become better clinicians while also seeing patients via telehealth. Marlene raises her two children in New Jersey and can be found on ball fields, beaches, or ski slopes in her spare time.

Array Behavioral Care, Mount Laurel, NJ, USA

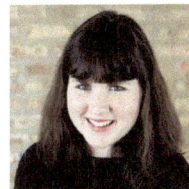

Bridget Mitchell is the Director of Clinical Operations for Compass Health Center. Prior to her work with Compass, Bridget was the Vice President of Scheduled Services for Array Behavioral Care (formerly InSight + Regroup), where she oversaw the operations, account management, and teleclinician engagement functions for telebehavioral partnerships at multiple clinical settings and healthcare systems across the United States. Her work with Array also included the development and standardization of telehealth operations and the creation of a clinician engagement program to support remotely located teleclinicians. Bridget earned her Master of Social Work degree from the University of Illinois at Chicago, with a concentration in Mental Health.

Compass Health Center, Northbrook, IL, USA

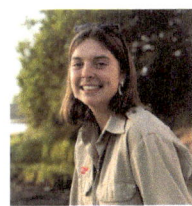

Emily Vogt is a medical student at the University of Michigan interested in telemedicine, innovation, and health equity research. Prior to medical school, Emily was an intramural research trainee at the National Institute on Alcohol Abuse and Alcoholism where she studied how psychosocial and genetic factors influence the etiology and treatment of alcohol use disorder. Emily is originally from Washington, DC, and completed her undergraduate degree in Neuroscience and Economics at Northwestern University. During her time as an undergraduate, she pursued an internship at a telehealth company in Chicago, which sparked her interest in telemedicine as a means to improve access to care and paved the way for several research projects and publications related to telebehavioral health. She currently lives in Ann Arbor with her partner where she enjoys exploring Michigan's abundance of parks and eclectic mix of restaurants.

Abbreviations

AACAP	American Academy of Child and Adolescent Psychiatry
ADHD	Attention deficit hyperactivity disorder
AI	Artificial intelligence
AIMS	Abnormal Involuntary Movement Scale
ACP	American College of Physicians
APA	American Psychiatric Association
ATA	American Telemedicine Association
ASL	American Sign Language
BAA	Business Associate Agreement
BH	Behavioral health
BHS	Behavioral health service(s)
CART	Communication Access Real-time Translation
cCBT	computerized cognitive behavioral therapy, synonym: Internet-based CBT or iCBT
CMS	Centers for Medicare and Medicaid Services
CoCM	Collaborative care model
CPT	Current procedural terminology
DEA	Drug Enforcement Agency
ED	Emergency department
EHR	Electronic health record(s)
EKG	Electrocardiogram
EPCS	Electronic Prescribing of Controlled Substances
FIPS	Federal Information Processing Standards
HIPAA	The Health Insurance Portability and Accountability Act

HITECH Act	The Health Information Technology for Economic and Clinical Health Act
HHS	The U.S. Department of Health & Human Services
HRQL	Health-Related Quality of Life
ICT	Information and communication technologies
IOP	Intensive outpatient program
IT	Information Technology
LGBTQ	Lesbian, gay, bisexual, transgender, and queer or questioning
M&E	Monitoring and Evaluation
MAR	Medication Administration Record
MAT	Medication-assisted treatment
MGH	Massachusetts General Hospital
PCP	Primary care provider
PHI	Protected health information
PROM	Patient-reported outcome measures
PSP	Patient Support Person
ROI	Release of information
OS	Originating site(s)
OUD	Opioid use disorder
PHP	Partial hospital program
PSP	Patient Support Person
PTSD	Post-Traumatic Stress Disorder
SDOH	Social determinants of health
SUD	Substance use disorder(s)
TBH	Telebehavioral health
WHO	World Health Organization

Introduction

Emile Whaibeh and Hossam Mahmoud

In the beginning was the chair, and the chair was reclined, and behind it sat the *man* with the notepad and the cigar, and he peered into the submerged part of the iceberg, asking questions about the childhood of the patient who laid down, staring at the moldy corners of the ceiling. Then, the *chaise longue* became smaller, grew sturdy arms, and became upright; the figure with the notepad, formerly out of the patient's sight, sat across from them, perched behind a wooden desk, listening intently until the exchange started to feel obstructed by the bulky table. So, they ditched the desk, each retiring into their own respective chairs, and they sat facing one another, communicating through verbal and nonverbal cues, seeking insight, clarity, and healthier coping skills.

Some days, the patient's chair lays empty. Perhaps they were held up at work or could not take the time or day off. Or perhaps they could not afford the transportation fees or the cost of the session. But there were other days when the chair also laid empty, yet the care continued, from a distance. At first, the patient might have just been a floor above or below, maybe even down the street. Later, they could be miles away, in different cities and across state

E. Whaibeh (✉)
Department of Public Health, Faculty of Health Sciences,
University of Balamand (UOB), Beirut, Lebanon

H. Mahmoud
Tufts University School of Medicine, Boston, MA, USA

H. Mahmoud et al. (eds.), *Essentials of Telebehavioral Health*,
https://doi.org/10.1007/978-3-030-97325-4_1

lines. Some patients were city dwellers; others lived in rural communities. Some were behind school walls, others behind bars. Regardless of where they were, who they were, how old they were, and what they needed, treatment always found new channels, harnessing the available technology of the time to bypass geographic constraints and usher the genesis of what is now widely known as telebehavioral health (TBH).

Simply put, TBH is the remote provision and delivery of mental health and substance use healthcare services using information and communication technologies (ICT). If you are not familiar with the term, you might have come across other terminology such as telepsychiatry, telepsychotherapy, telemental health, or virtual behavioral health. Other terms used when referring to TBH also include electronic health (e-health), mobile health (m-health), and digital health. While every term conveys some nuances, these terms have, to some extent, been used interchangeably in peer-reviewed literature and among healthcare organizations. For consistency, this book will use the term TBH. The value of TBH has been recognized for several decades and its adoption had been gradually increasing for several years, with somewhat accelerated adoption between 2015 and 2019. This was due to the increase in demand for BHS, improvements in hardware and software technology, expanded broadband Internet and connectivity, and the growing research supporting the effectiveness and acceptance of TBH.

Then, in 2020, the world was taken by a storm that would prove hard to weather. On March 11 of that year, the World Health Organization (WHO) declared Coronavirus Disease 2019 (COVID-19) a pandemic [1]. While some experts had warned about the possibility of a pandemic, few could have predicted the devastating impact of this global disease on every facet of our lives. The tidal waves of the pandemic dramatically disrupted the delivery of healthcare services, forcing institutions to promptly transform to adapt. This transformation was prompted by multiple factors: concerns about exposure to the virus, physical distance directives, and varying degrees of lockdown. This was accompanied by an increase in the incidence and prevalence of behavioral health (BH) conditions and demand for behavioral health services

(BHS), which some dubbed as the "pandemic within the pandemic" [2]. This BH pandemic, manifesting in increased rates of anxiety, mood and substance use disorders, among other symptoms, is yet to be fully understood. It has been attributed to several factors, including the stress caused by COVID-19 itself, reported psychiatric symptoms post-recovery from the infection, lockdowns, physical distancing safety measures, and the economic downturn [3]. At the time of writing this book, it remains unclear how long and to what extent we will be reeling from the long-term BH consequences.

To go back to our patient–clinician duo, the chair, once more, lies empty, or *lay* empty, depending on where you are and how much the situation is under control by the time you have picked up this book. Regardless of where we stand vis-à-vis the COVID-19 pandemic, its effect on the BHS landscape is potentially irreversible. Clinicians and healthcare institutions, as you are well aware by now, found themselves forced to adapt to the *new normal* and transition into TBH or different variations of hybrid in-person and virtual models. Due to concerns about exposure, physical distancing measures, clinical safety, or simply clinician or patient preference, TBH became the primary, if not the only, option to meet the needs of their patients in a rapidly evolving pandemic. TBH adoption was also facilitated by a range of regulatory changes introduced by federal and state governments across the United States, and concomitant reimbursement changes by payers. These included executive orders requiring parity in payment for TBH services as in-person BHS, suspending some cross-state licensure requirements, and lifting certain restrictions on remote prescribing, to name a few.

Sure enough, the public health emergency was a catalyst that fueled a digital health revolution that had been gaining momentum for the past decade. By April 2020, the United States witnessed a 50% increase in telemedicine use on a national level [4]. Similarly, a physician survey in the United States found that 48% of physicians were using telemedicine in some capacity in 2020 compared to just 18% of physicians 2 years prior [5]. With 41.1% of US adults reporting symptoms of anxiety disorder and depression in January 2021, according to the National Center for Health

Statistics and the U.S. Census Bureau's Household Pulse Survey, TBH is poised to achieve even more growth in years to come [6]. It is no coincidence that investors over the last 2 years have channeled millions of dollars into platforms and startups that deliver, enable, or facilitate the delivery of TBH services.

Yet, we are creatures of habit. This is a safe space to admit that readjusting and re-evaluating one's clinical practices to accommodate a "new" modality can feel at the very least overwhelming, especially against a backdrop of ever-expanding and rapidly changing BHS landscape. If you are a BH clinician, then you are aware of the gradual shift of the historical clinical space, with strategically placed couches and chairs, indoor plants, and neutral paintings, over decades. The pandemic has precipitously disrupted and eroded the frame you always tried to hold during a session [7]. But whether you run a private practice or manage a healthcare institution, the COVID-19 pandemic created a watershed moment to adapt one's services and clinical practices to meet patient needs.

If you are reading this book, you have either already made the transition from in-person care to hybrid or completely virtual care, or you might have just gotten started and need some guidance, or you are still somewhat skeptical about TBH but still fairly interested in making the transition. No matter where you stand on that spectrum, you will find, after a quick literature search, that there is an abundance of peer-reviewed journal articles and publications documenting the efficacy, cost-efficiency, and clinical benefits of TBH, many even dating back to a pre-COVID-19 period. However, there are few standardized frameworks in place for conceptualizing, planning, implementing, and evaluating TBH programs, and even fewer that do so in a condensed yet succinct fashion.

Essentials of Telebehavioral Health—A Practical Guide is a user-friendly companion for clinicians and other healthcare professionals looking for practical guidance in setting up and maintaining TBH practices. The book provides clinical, operational, regulatory, and technical guidance on TBH, based on robust literature review and the authors' and editors' experience in researching, planning, implementing, delivering, and monitoring

TBH programs across multiple clinical settings. We recognize that there is a wide range of TBH care delivery models, for direct care and consultation, including synchronous and asynchronous communication through multiple text, audio, and video-based platforms. While we do make reference to the various approaches, this book focuses primarily on the delivery of direct patient care delivered in a synchronous manner between two parties, the tele-clinician and the patient, via videoconferencing, as this continues to constitute the primary approach to delivering TBH services.

Essentials of Telebehavioral Health breaks TBH down to its basics, condensing its seemingly intimidating and overwhelming aspects down to a handful of essential components represented by the acronym "OPTIC" (see Fig. 1.1) to serve as a foundation for discussing TBH programs.

"OPTIC" refers to the five core components of any TBH program or practice that involves direct patient care. (O) stands for the "originating site," and it refers to the brick-and-mortar location where the patient receives services. This could be a private clinic, healthcare facility, community health center, hospital,

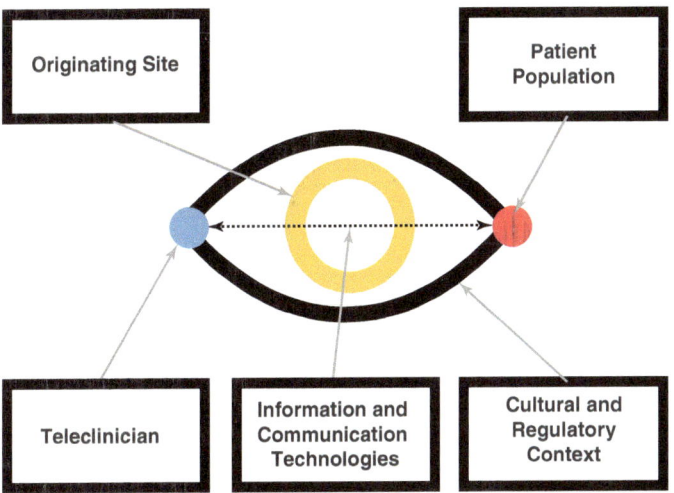

Fig. 1.1 The OPTIC acronym of core components of any TBH practice

school, university health center, correctional facility, or patient's home. (P) stands for the "patient" or the "patient population," and it refers to the individual or individuals who are receiving BHS remotely. (T) refers to "teleclinician" and includes healthcare professional(s) providing BHS remotely. Note that the teleclinician's location is typically referred to as the "distant site," although it can also be referred to as the provider or physician site or consulting site [8]. (I) refers to "information and communication technologies," and it includes both the software and hardware used to deliver care remotely, including videoconferencing platforms and other communication methods used between teleclinicians and patients and between teleclinicians and other healthcare professionals. ICT can also include web-based applications, smartphone applications, electronic health record systems, and electronic prescribing systems. Finally, (C) stands for the "cultural and regulatory context" 'that shape and govern the delivery of TBH services.

The book is divided into nine chapters in addition to a resource section toward the end. Chapter 2 covers the basics of TBH as well as a history of its evolution since the 1950s. Chapters 3–7 cover the OPTIC components, with one chapter dedicated to every component. Chapter 8 covers monitoring, evaluation, and quality assurance for TBH programs. Finally, Chapter 9 discusses current trends and anticipated directions that TBH will likely evolve into in the future.

While this work serves as a practical guide to delivering TBH services, it should be considered in the context of the ever-evolving regulatory variations that shape the delivery of BHS, in general, and TBH, in particular. It is still imperative that clinicians and program directors familiarize themselves with the laws and regulations in the jurisdictions where the patient population is located, the policies of their organizations and healthcare facilities, and the updated best practices and care standards published by professional societies.

Finally, in writing *Essentials of Telebehavioral Health*, the authors and editors hope to support the delivery of high-quality, well-informed, and culturally appropriate TBH services to help expand access to BHS, overcome barriers to care, and ultimately decrease healthcare disparities.

References

1. World Health Organization. WHO Director-General's opening remarks at the media briefing on COVID-19-11 March 2020. World Health Organization; 2020. https://www.who.int/director-general/speeches/detail/who-director-general-s-opening-remarks-at-the-media-briefing-on-covid-19%2D%2D-11-march-2020. Accessed June 3, 2021.

2. Qureshi S. Pandemics within the pandemic: confronting socio-economic inequities in a datafied world. Inf Technol Dev. 2021; https://doi.org/10.1080/02681102.2021.1911020.

3. Whaibeh E, Mahmoud H, Naal H. Telemental health in the context of a pandemic: the COVID-19 experience. Curr Treat Options Psychiatry. https://doi.org/10.1007/s40501-020-00210-2.

4. Koonin LM, Hoots B, Tsang CA, Leroy Z, Farris K, Jolly BT, Antal P, McCabe B, Zelis CBR, Tong I, Harris AM. Trends in the use of telehealth during the emergence of the COVID-10 pandemic - United States, January-March 2020. Morb Mortal Wkly Rep. 2020;69(43):1595–9.

5. Merritt Hawkins. Survey: physician practice patterns changing as a result of COVID-19. Merritt Hawkins; 2020. https://www.merritthawkins.com/news-and-insights/media-room/press/-physician-practice-patterns-changing-as-a-result-of-covid-19/. Accessed 3 June 2021.

6. Panchal N, Kamal R, Cox C, Garfield R. The implications of COVID-19 for mental health and substance use. Kaiser Family Foundation; 2021. https://www.kff.org/report-section/the-implications-of-covid-19-for-mental-health-and-substance-use-issue-brief/. Accessed 3 June 2021.

7. Gopnik A. The new theatrics of remote therapy: how does treatment change when your patients are on a screen? Coronavirus Chronicles. The New Yorker. 2020. https://www.newyorker.com/magazine/2020/06/01/the-new-theatrics-of-remote-therapy. Accessed 3 June 2021.

8. Board on Health Care Services, Institute of Medicine. The role of Telehealth in an evolving health care environment: workshop summary. Washington (DC): National Academies Press (US). 2012. Appendix A, Definitions. https://www.ncbi.nlm.nih.gov/books/NBK207151/. Accessed 3 June 2021.

Telebehavioral Health: The Basics

2

Emily Vogt and Emile Whaibeh

Telebehavioral health (TBH) is the use of information and communication technologies (ICT), including but not limited to videoconferencing, to remotely deliver behavioral health services (BHS). While this is the most widely accepted definition, TBH has evolved with the advances in ICT and models of healthcare delivery, and the more "traditional" definition of two-way live videoconferencing has expanded to incorporate digital self-navigated modules, asynchronous care delivery, smartphone applications, and different consultative models. This has led to the use of some terms such as electronic health (e-health), mobile health (m-health), and digital health under the umbrella of TBH. As mentioned in Chap. 1, while recognizing the utility of different approaches to delivering virtual BHS, this book focuses primarily on the delivery of direct patient care via videoconferencing in a synchronous manner between two parties, the teleclinician and the patient.

E. Vogt
University of Michigan Medical School, Ann Arbor, MI, USA
e-mail: vogtem@med.umich.edu

E. Whaibeh (✉)
Department of Public Health, Faculty of Health Sciences, University of Balamand (UOB), Beirut, Lebanon

© The Author(s), under exclusive license to Springer Nature Switzerland AG 2022
H. Mahmoud et al. (eds.), *Essentials of Telebehavioral Health*, https://doi.org/10.1007/978-3-030-97325-4_2

9

Because of its seeming novelty and its use of sophisticated ICT, it might come as a surprise for some readers to learn that TBH has existed in different forms and capacities since the 1950s, which is to say that TBH is actually older than the World Wide Web. The purpose of this chapter is to familiarize the reader with key TBH concepts, the range of TBH services, TBH advantages and challenges, and a brief history of its evolution, contextualizing its development.

TBH Services

TBH has been used to deliver a wide range of BHS encompassing the continuum of needs, including health promotion, prevention, treatment, and recovery services. Accordingly, TBH can be used to treat mental health and substance use disorders (SUDs), provide emotional support, and promote mental well-being. TBH services can include psychiatric evaluations, medication management, psychotherapy, psychoeducation, consultation services, and self-navigated digital modules [1, 2].

TBH programs have often been deployed to improve care availability, reduce long patient wait-times, and access a wider and more diverse pool of clinicians in the context of the national shortage and uneven distribution of BH clinicians [3]. For patients with limited capacity to travel due to physical limitations, transportation challenges, cost limitations, or time constraints, TBH significantly helps in mitigating barriers to care by eliminating or minimizing the need for patients to travel in order to receive BHS. This advantage also applies to patients struggling with certain mental health conditions that limit their ability to travel such as agoraphobia, severe depression, post-traumatic stress disorder (PTSD), or social anxiety [3, 4]. Furthermore, TBH can address the needs of a wide range of patient populations and treatment needs, and it can be delivered by a wide range of clinicians such as psychiatrists, psychiatric advanced practice nurses, psychologists, and social workers [5].

Dubbed as a "disruptive innovation," TBH has been changing the landscape of healthcare delivery [6], even before the

COVID-19 pandemic. In recent years, it underwent significant growth [7], which was aided by several factors, including (1) increased high-speed Internet connectivity and availability of ICT software and hardware, (2) increased acceptability of TBH among both patients and clinicians, (3) expanded reimbursement models, and (4) increased demand for BHS paired with the inability of healthcare systems to meet the BH needs of the population [8].

TBH adoption was further catapulted by the COVID-19 pandemic due to the need to prioritize hospital space for COVID-19 patients, the health risks posed by in-person visits, and the lockdown measures that drove many healthcare institutions to utilize remote healthcare delivery whenever feasible [9, 10]. Indeed, the data reveal an unprecedented increase in TBH utilization: the Veterans Affairs Health Administration reported more than 300 million virtual video visits in June 2020 alone, an 11-fold increase from the previous five months [11]. Additionally, a study with tele-psychologists indicated that, on average, more than 85% of their clinical practice during COVID-19 was done remotely, a more than 12-fold increase from the pre-pandemic period [12].

TBH utilizes different approaches to care delivery, including synchronous and asynchronous services. Synchronous services are those delivered in real time and are the main focus of this book. They encompass most of the direct patient care TBH services, largely occurring via live two-way videoconferencing. In contrast, asynchronous services use store and forward ICT in the form of video messages, audio messages, email, and messaging applications to deliver services in a manner that is not in real time [2, 13]. Currently, asynchronous services are used to deliver a wide range of services, including direct patient care and consultation services [2, 13]. Not only do asynchronous TBH services help improve access to care in a cost-efficient manner but they also offer improved convenience for clinicians and patients, eliminating the need for appointments and concomitant scheduling "friction" [14]. When advantageous to serving institutional and patient needs, TBH programs can follow a hybrid model of synchronous and asynchronous TBH, aimed at improving system-wide access to care in different clinical settings [13]. In addition, with advances in ICT, particularly smartphone applications, there has been an expansion of digital health services to deliver support through self-guided modules targeting resilience, coping with stress, insomnia, depressive symptoms, anxiety symptoms, among others. These modules aim to address milder conditions and BH symptoms or to complement other more direct approaches for BHS delivery. They often employ computerized cognitive behavioral therapy (cCBT) or other evidence-based psychotherapy approaches, and they are sometimes supported with personalized coaching to improve engagement and utilization.

The Evolution of Telebehavioral Health in the United States

The following section offers a brief overview of the history and evolution of TBH through the decades, along with the various applications that have shaped its trajectory (see Fig. 2.1).

The Pioneering Experiments

In the mid-1950s, growing concern about the overcrowding and understaffing of "mental hospitals" in the United States generally, and in California particularly, motivated the superintendent and medical director of Agnews State Hospital, Hyman Tucker, to explore new ways to deliver BHS. The aim was to provide "mass therapy" that reaches a large number of patients in a cost-effective way. As such, an experiment was conducted in 1954 with a group of 141 "psychotic women patients." The experimental group ($n = 66$) was exposed to both commercial broadcast and closed-circuit television therapeutic sessions while the control group ($n = 75$) was exposed to commercial broadcast only. It was found that therapy by closed-circuit television significantly improved the behavioral patterns of patients in areas like communication, interpersonal relationships, socialization, and self-care [15]. Despite being a pioneering experiment, the Agnews State Hospital experiment does not often receive a lot of attention in the literature by virtue of it being a single rudimentary study with no programmatic follow-up.

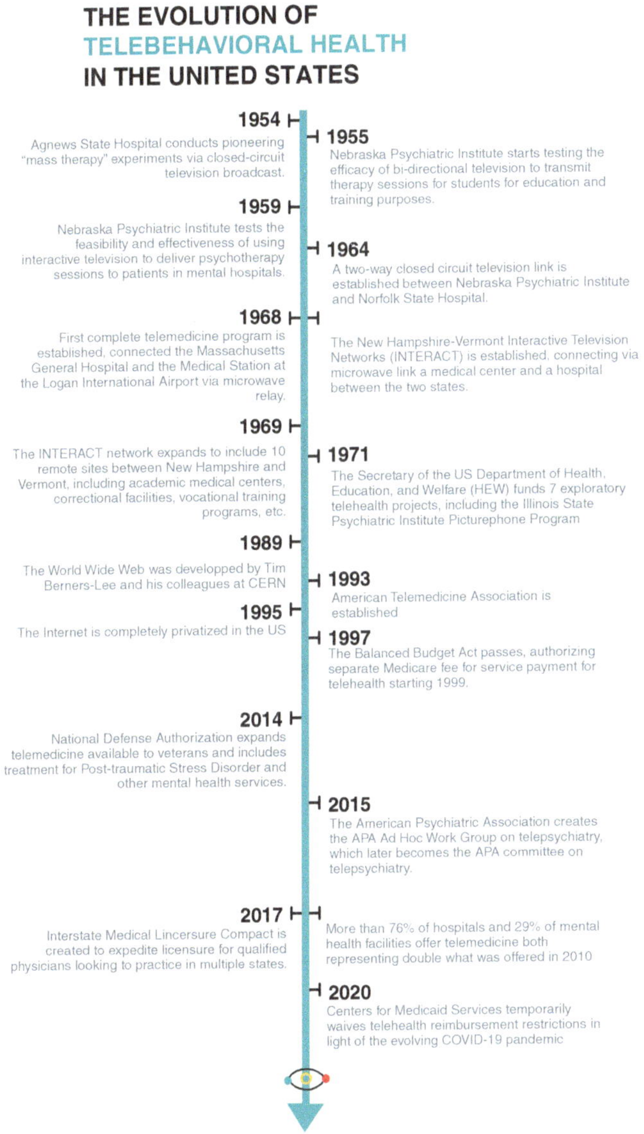

THE EVOLUTION OF
TELEBEHAVIORAL HEALTH
IN THE UNITED STATES

1954
Agnews State Hospital conducts pioneering "mass therapy" experiments via closed-circuit television broadcast.

1955
Nebraska Psychiatric Institute starts testing the efficacy of bi-directional television to transmit therapy sessions for students for education and training purposes.

1959
Nebraska Psychiatric Institute tests the feasibility and effectiveness of using interactive television to deliver psychotherapy sessions to patients in mental hospitals.

1964
A two-way closed circuit television link is established between Nebraska Psychiatric Institute and Norfolk State Hospital.

1968
First complete telemedicine program is established, connected the Massachusetts General Hospital and the Medical Station at the Logan International Airport via microwave relay.

The New Hampshire-Vermont Interactive Television Networks (INTERACT) is established, connecting via microwave link a medical center and a hospital between the two states.

1969
The INTERACT network expands to include 10 remote sites between New Hampshire and Vermont, including academic medical centers, correctional facilities, vocational training programs, etc.

1971
The Secretary of the US Department of Health, Education, and Welfare (HEW) funds 7 exploratory telehealth projects, including the Illinois State Psychiatric Institute Picturephone Program

1989
The World Wide Web was developped by Tim Berners-Lee and his colleagues at CERN

1993
American Telemedicine Association is established

1995
The Internet is completely privatized in the US

1997
The Balanced Budget Act passes, authorizing separate Medicare fee for service payment for telehealth starting 1999.

2014
National Defense Authorization expands telemedicine available to veterans and includes treatment for Post-traumatic Stress Disorder and other mental health services.

2015
The American Psychiatric Association creates the APA Ad Hoc Work Group on telepsychiatry, which later becomes the APA committee on telepsychiatry.

2017
Interstate Medical Lincersure Compact is created to expedite licensure for qualified physicians looking to practice in multiple states.

More than 76% of hospitals and 29% of mental health facilities offer telemedicine both representing double what was offered in 2010

2020
Centers for Medicaid Services temporarily waives telehealth reimbursement restrictions in light of the evolving COVID-19 pandemic

Fig. 2.1 Timeline of the evolution of telebehavioral health in the United States

For some, the history of TBH started around the same time over 1000 miles away from the Golden State in Omaha, Nebraska. In 1955, Dr. Cecil Wittson of the Nebraska Psychiatric Institute started testing the feasibility of bidirectional television to transmit therapy sessions for students, primarily for educational and training purposes [16]. These experiments proved to be successful, which prompted the development of other applications, enabling professionals from the Psychiatry Department to interact with colleagues in other related disciplines. Even though the initial experiments were conducted between close locations, Dr. Wittson reasoned that once these applications were extended over longer distances, they would enable remote clinical interactions between psychiatrists and other medical specialists in a time-efficient and cost-effective way [17]. In 1959, Wittson and his colleagues tested the feasibility and effectiveness of using interactive television to deliver group psychotherapy sessions to patients in "mental hospitals." The study found no difference between the experimental group, which received therapy via a two-way television, and the control group, which received therapy in person. This finding suggested that the medium of delivery had no effect, and therefore, traditional therapy could be replaced by its televised counterpart [18]. Based on these experiments, an operational telepsychiatry program was established in Nebraska in 1964. The two-way closed-circuit television link was the first of its kind, and it connected the Nebraska Psychiatric Institute in Omaha to the Norfolk State Hospital, located 112 miles away [18].

In 1968, after 4 years of planning, the first complete prototype telemedicine program was established in Boston. It provided a range of primary care and emergency services, including psychiatric services, to the employees, workers, and travelers at Logan International Airport. The program connected the Medical Station at the airport to Massachusetts General Hospital (MGH) via microwave relay [17]. Between 1968 and 1970, a total of 1400 patients at the Logan Medical Station were seen virtually by specialists at MGH [17]. The visits were assisted by the presence of a nurse at the Medical Station. During the first two years of its deployment, the program offered psychiatric consultations to 150 patients, some of whom received further follow-up visits. MGH then expanded their telepsychiatry services to junior high schools, a municipal court, a department of corrections on a nearby island, and a Veterans Administration Psychiatric Hospital in Bedford, Massachusetts [17]. Based on this experiment, psychiatric consultations via interactive television ensured more privacy for patients and were found to be easier for some patients "than contact in the same room." This sentiment was especially true for patients with schizophrenia, as well as children and adolescents with behavioral problems [19].

Around the same time, in 1968, a two-way television microwave link, known as the New Hampshire-Vermont Medical Interactive Television Network or "INTERACT," was established between the Hitchcock Hospital at the Dartmouth Medical Center, Hanover, New Hampshire, and Claremont General Hospital, Vermont. It was the first telemedicine program linking two healthcare institutions in two neighboring states [17]. In the following year, the program expanded further, following a hub-and-spoke design whereby Dartmouth Medical School served as the hub facility, connected through microwave transmission to 10 remote sites in various locations in New Hampshire and Vermont. The sites included academic medical centers, correctional facilities, and vocational training programs [17]. The goal of the program was to offer ongoing medical education for healthcare professionals, remote specialty medical services in the fields of psychiatry, oncology, dermatology, and speech therapy, when such services were unavailable at the local community level. Finally, the program provided training and capacity-building for healthcare staff to promote the sharing of professional responsibilities and meeting the health needs of the population in rural New England. Despite diversifying their services, the network was mostly used for educational purposes and for consultations among physicians; it is estimated that direct patient care made up only 10% of the program [17].

The "Coming-of-Age" Period

The period between 1972 and 1980 witnessed such a great gain in momentum for telemedicine in the United States that it was dubbed the "coming of age era of telemedicine" [17]. Several factors contributed to the increased interest in providing remote healthcare services, including BHS. First, the previously mentioned programs in Nebraska, Massachusetts, New Hampshire, and Vermont yielded promising positive results; these pioneering programs showed great potential and effectiveness in improving access to BHS for underserved patients and providing educational opportunities for students and healthcare professionals. Second, the manned space program of the National Aeronautics and Space Administration (NASA) was receiving a lot of attention for its achievements, including the less-discussed role in the development and deployment of telemedicine technology to ensure the health, safety, and well-being of astronauts. Finally, the United States still needed solutions to grave challenges that were facing healthcare systems, with limited access to care for certain segments of the population, uneven geographic distribution of healthcare services, and increased health costs.

In light of these conditions, the federal government supported research and development in the field of telemedicine with the rationale of harnessing advances in communication technology to improve the access of the American people to quality BHS while limiting the growing cost of care. Following the call for proposals made in 1971 by the Secretary of The US Department of Health, Education, and Welfare (HEW), seven exploratory projects (out of 22 that applied) were selected to receive a first-year budget of $1,158,056 each. Out of the seven projects, the Illinois State Psychiatric Institute Picturephone Program was the only one exclusively dedicated to BHS. The aim of the program was to explore the utility of two-way visual communication for paramedical personnel found in clinics to receive expert consultations from medical experts found in hospitals or other clinics nearby. To achieve that, the Illinois State Psychiatric Institute was made into a hub connected to several satellite locations: the Illinois State

Pediatric Institute, located one city block away, the Health School, located two blocks away, the Institute for Juvenile Research and the West Side Organizations, found three blocks away, and the Pilsen Community Center, located one mile away. Satellite locations were located in low-income neighborhoods on the west side of Chicago. As the name of the program indicates, the adopted technology of choice was the Picturephone, a two-way video communication device that uses telephone circuits, analog black-and-white video transmission similar to television broadcasting of the time, and a $5'' \times 5.5''$ screen [20].

The Illinois Program faced several shortcomings, starting with the prohibitive cost of the Picturephone technology and their inability to demonstrate the clinical effectiveness and the cost-efficiency of telemedicine. Moreover, even though over the years healthcare personnel in satellite locations were increasingly utilizing the Picturephone to consult medical experts and to attend hospital conferences and training sessions remotely, the Illinois Program could not ultimately sustain itself without federal funding. The Illinois Program and the other federally funded projects had to (1) identify the appropriate technology and needed infrastructure, (2) estimate future utilization of the offered services, and (3) establish cost-effective communication and transportation networks in diverse settings. The governing bodies overseeing the projects underestimated the difficulty of these tasks, and the mounting political pressure pushed them to rush through these three stages into one in order to demonstrate as quickly as possible positive results to justify the federal spending; this contributed to the unfortunate failure of these programs [17].

While the 1970s were marked by great optimism and faith in the promise of TBH, the decade also witnessed the discontinuance of the Illinois Program, the 6 other federally funded programs, and 11 other telemedicine programs funded by different sources. Also, despite differences in geographic locations, special populations served, and services provided, all telemedicine programs of the era met similar fates. Not only were they unable to remain operational without external funding but they also could not provide skeptics and policymakers with sufficient evidence on the effectiveness and cost-efficiency of telemedicine. However, as

Preston et al. [21] remarked, a significant challenge for a lot of those programs was poor system management as reporting structures were blurred and responsibilities were sometimes unclear. Despite this major setback, the advocates of telemedicine were not dissuaded, even if the field came to a gradual halt in the early 1980s. It would take until the end of the decade for new state-based initiatives to begin establishing strong TBH networks within states.

The Resurgence of TBH in the 1990s

The 1990s brought a notable surge in utilization of TBH. This period was marked by the launch and consistent growth of large and sustained TBH programs [22], facilitated by several factors. First, ICT became more available and affordable, which enhanced access, familiarity, and usability of hardware and software needed to participate in telehealth sessions. Second, the Internet, introduced in 1989, became completely privatized in 1995; this led to newly offered affordable plans and services that gave more people access to the World Wide Web. While only 14% of US adults had Internet access in 1995, and most were using slow dial-up modems, the introduction of the Internet to healthcare settings allowed healthcare personnel to share medical documents (such as X-rays, scans, vital signs, electrocardiograms [EKG]) and allowed for real-time audiovisual communication [23]. Third, large-scale TBH programs were deployed within larger systems and institutions such as correctional facilities, universities, and federal health systems [24]. These systems proved to be more sustainable as they served large patient populations and benefited from the cost reduction of ICT [22]. Fourth, in 1993, the American Telemedicine Association (ATA), a nonprofit organization focused on enhancing access to care by accelerating the adoption of telehealth, was founded [25]. In order to educate and increase the acceptability of remote healthcare services for both policymakers and the general public, the ATA, through its Standards and Guidelines Committee, developed quality-of-care guidelines for remote services, including TBH services, with the Telemental

Health Practice Guideline being one of their most commonly downloaded documents [25]. Finally, the Balanced Budget Act of 1997 was the pivotal event that catapulted the expansion of telemedicine, which occurred toward the end of the decade, and which authorized separate Medicare Fee For Service payment for telehealth starting 1999. This set the tone for the whole country and was a precursor for Medicaid and other payers to start reimbursing for TBH services thereafter [26].

The 2000s and Beyond

In the 2000s, TBH adoption and the scientific literature supporting its safety, cost-effectiveness, and efficacy continued to grow [3]. In addition, from 2000 until 2014, the percentage of adults in the United States who used the Internet increased from 52% to 84% [27]. The introduction and widespread availability of multiple web-based videoconferencing programs meant that people were becoming increasingly familiar with the technology. This also created a shift in TBH delivery because programs and teleclinicians were no longer restricted to traditional clinical settings to deliver care since it became possible to deliver care into patients' homes or offices. Meanwhile, legislative attempts to regulate online pharmacies led to the passing of the Ryan Haight Online Pharmacy Consumer Protection Act of 2008. This act ended up having an unintended yet significant impact on regulating and limiting the prescribing of controlled substances through TBH [28], as will be discussed in Chap. 7.

TBH services were increasingly offered by private clinicians, as well as a growing number of TBH organizations [29]. Private practices, community health centers, and hospital systems began deploying and adopting TBH services [22]. From 2010 to 2017, the percentage of hospitals in the United States providing telemedicine for their patients increased from 35% to 76% [30]. As for BH facilities, the percentage of facilities offering TBH nearly doubled from 1580 (15.2% of all facilities) in 2010 to 3385 (29.2% of all facilities) in 2017 [31, 32]. TBH started attracting more attention and interest in investment as the technology sector grew rapidly, with increased demand for TBH services. Startups and other healthcare technology companies began to develop TBH programs for both healthcare clinics and patients in need of BHS.

More recently, in the face of the COVID-19 pandemic, healthcare providers increasingly resorted to using TBH services to avoid disruptions to care delivery, while following public safety preventative measures of social distancing. On the reimbursement front, the Centers for Medicare & Medicaid Services (CMS) waived geographic and originating site (OS) restrictions for telehealth, including TBH, during the crisis, thus allowing for Medicare reimbursement regardless of patient location [26]. In addition, executive orders and legislations in several jurisdictions were passed during the pandemic to expand or require coverage of telehealth services, sometimes at parity.

As for investments in the health technology industry, venture capital funding funneled to health technology innovators exceeded US$14 billion in 2020, twice as much as in 2019, and they are projected to continue to grow [33].

The Evolving Role of TBH

The marked expansion of TBH in the past decade, specifically following the COVID-19 pandemic, illustrates the evolving role that TBH will play in BHS delivery. The growing body of research and implementation reports has been instrumental to TBH's growth, both in validating its efficacy as a care delivery method and in exploring its operationalization across a range of clinical models and settings. In this section, we discuss some advantages and challenges that have been identified for TBH, to provide further context prior to discussing the OPTIC components.

Despite the historical skepticism TBH faced, there is strong evidence in support of its effectiveness across a wide range of contexts in terms of both clinical and nonclinical outcomes [2, 3]. Patient engagement and satisfaction have been the most commonly used nonclinical measures to assess TBH programs, while standardized clinical scales have been commonly used to assess TBH efficacy on clinical outcomes [34]. TBH has performed strongly across both clinical and nonclinical measures, proving to be equivalent and in some cases superior to in-person care in terms of patient satisfaction, patient follow-up, wait-time, and clinical improvement [2, 3, 34, 35]. Importantly, TBH does not appear to compromise the therapeutic alliance and, in some respects, can create a more comfortable setting for patients, which can then facilitate better patient–clinician rapport-building [36, 37].

Additional studies have validated the utility of TBH across a wide range of more specific clinical contexts, diagnoses, ages, and patient populations, each with their own implementation-related nuances. TBH has been shown to have useful applications across academic medical centers, community health clinics, critical access hospitals, correctional facilities, residential-based healthcare programs, and within First Nations communities [38]. Within and across these settings, there is substantial evidence that TBH is an effective means of delivering care across a broad spectrum of populations and diagnoses, including but not limited to attention-deficit hyperactivity disorder (ADHD), depression, anxiety, schizophrenia, PTSD, SUD, suicide prevention, eating disorders, dementia, and mental health concerns related to movement disorders [39].

Beyond its comparative efficacy to in-person interventions, TBH also presents several specific advantages that make it an especially useful tool. First, TBH expands access to care. While this point became particularly cogent during the COVID-19 pandemic when TBH became the only option for care delivery for many, this fact holds true even when in-person care delivery is possible. For instance, TBH has been particularly impactful in rural areas, where patients who might not be able to travel long distances are able to access specialists from the comfort of their homes [2, 3, 9]. Additionally, TBH has a strong potential in addressing historic gaps associated with BH care delivery to rural communities, where it is particularly challenging to recruit and retain psychiatrists [40]. A recent analysis of Medicare claims data shows that telehealth is most frequently utilized by rural healthcare providers affiliated with larger hospital groups or healthcare systems, possibly to allow these clinicians to serve rural communities without being completely isolated from academic activities or professional support [41].

In addition to transcending geographic barriers associated with access to behavioral healthcare, TBH also can help in overcoming stigma barriers associated with accessing BHS [40]. TBH allows patients to seek care from the comfort of their homes, thereby reducing the social ramifications associated with being seen at a BHS clinic and mitigating patients' fear of lack of acceptance in certain treatment settings [42]. This advantage may be especially relevant in cultural contexts that stigmatize BH conditions or that stigmatize seeking care for such conditions, such as SUD. TBH has also proven advantageous in delivering culturally appropriate care for underserved and marginalized populations, such as Lesbian, Gay, Bisexual, Transgender, and Queer (LGBTQ) patients who face many challenges accessing LGBTQ appropriate care [42, 43].

Financially, TBH has been shown to reduce direct and indirect healthcare costs due to several factors such as eliminating opportunity cost associated with travel time, eliminating the cost of travel, improving and facilitating continuity of care, and providing earlier interventions. While implementation of TBH does require some upfront costs that can vary depending on the existing technological infrastructure and workforce at a given site [44], creative, cost-balancing approaches, such as expanding patient volume via telehealth, using hybrid models of synchronous and asynchronous care and incorporating integrated consultative models can offer a potentially more sustainable model for implementation [13, 45]. Additionally, the COVID-19 pandemic has initiated an ongoing conversation amongst payers about continuing to reimburse for certain telehealth-based visits, which has the potential to make TBH an even more cost-effective intervention than it was prior to the pandemic [46].

Certainly, TBH has faced some challenges in its expansion. Certain clinical limitations have been identified in the literature. Aspects of a patient's presentation such as body language, non-verbal cues, and mild intoxication may be more difficult to pick up over video for certain patients, and there may be limitations in assessing physical exam components that are necessary for certain contexts [47, 48]. That said, this limitation can be overcome in facility-based TBH programs through the support of telehealth navigators, nurses, and other on-site staff. Another challenge is that TBH largely depends on access to technology and reliable Internet connection. While ICT have become more accessible and less costly, there are still many under-resourced areas and patient populations that lack access to these technologies. Even for those that do have access to technology, variable Internet connection affecting the quality of the videoconferencing experience can be a frequently cited frustration of virtual visits [48].

Other challenges to TBH have historically been the lack of formal training and limited staffing. Prior to the COVID-19 pandemic, few training programs for medical students, clinical psychology trainees, or residents incorporated formal TBH education and training [48, 49]. Moreover, while having dedicated staff to help manage TBH-related workflows has been demonstrated to significantly improve their adoption and sustainability, these positions have often been overlooked during program development and implementation due to attributed costs and underestimation of importance [1, 50].

Finally, cost remains a challenge to TBH program expansion and sustainability. Despite TBH's ability to be cost-effective or cost-saving in certain situations, as discussed above, restrictive guidelines related to reimbursement for TBH services, coupled with hefty start-up costs for program implementation, have limited wider-scale adoption of TBH across the country [44, 48]. Reimbursement has been a notoriously complex process for TBH, with numerous restrictions related to patient and teleclinician location, healthcare facility type, and lack of uniformity in reimbursement across payers and Medicaid programs [48]. However, as a result of the COVID-19 pandemic, private and public payers have temporarily relaxed these restrictions, and there is hope for improved reimbursement going forward that may improve the cost-efficacy of TBH programs [9, 51].

Despite the challenges, TBH has become a recognized cornerstone of healthcare systems and will continue to play a significant role in reshaping the landscape of healthcare delivery and improving access to care. We hope that this overview of the literature has provided some context on the historical progression of TBH, along with its wide range of applications. Given the flexibility and spectrum of TBH care, the subsequent chapters will discuss the OPTIC components of TBH programs in detail to guide you through the planning, implementation, and evaluation processes of your TBH program.

References

1. Mahmoud H, Whaibeh E, Mitchel B. Ensuring successful telepsychiatry program implementation: critical components and considerations. Curr Treatment Opt Psychiatry. 2020;7:186–97.

2. Langarizadeh M, Tabatabaei MS, Tavakol K, Naghipour M, Rostami A, Moghbeli F. Telemental health care, an effective alternative to conventional mental care: a systematic review. Acta Informatica Medica. 2017;25(4):240–6.

3. Hilty DM, Ferrer DC, Parish MB, Johnston B, Callahan EJ, Yellowlees PM. The effectiveness of telemental health: a 2013 review. Telemedicine e-Health. 2013;19(6):444–54.

4. APA. APA and ATA release new telemental health guide. American Psychiatric Association; 2018.

5. Maheu MM, Drude KP, Hertlein KM, Hilty DM. A framework of interprofessional telebehavioral health competencies: implementation and challenges moving forward. Acad Psychiatry. 2018;42(6):825–33.

6. Yellowlees P, Odor A, Patrice K, Parish M, Nafiz N, Losif A-M, et al. Disruptive innovation: the future of healthcare? Telemedicine e-Health. 2011;17(3):231–4.

7. Spivak S, Spivak A, Cullen B, Meuchel J, Johnston D, Chernow R, et al. Telepsychiatry use in U.S. Mental Health Facilities, 2010–2017. Psychiatric Services. 2019;appi.ps.2019002.

8. Mahmoud H, Vogt EL, Dahdouh R, Raymond ML. Using continuous quality improvement to design and implement a telepsychiatry program in rural Illinois. Psychiatr Serv 2020;appi.ps.2019002.

9. Shore JH, Schneck CD, Mishkind MC. Telepsychiatry and the coronavirus disease 2019 pandemic-current and future outcomes of the rapid virtualization of psychiatric care. JAMA. 2020;77:1211–2.

10. Augusterfer EF, O'Neal CR, Martin SW, Sheikh TL, Mollica RF. The role of telemental health, tele-consultation, and tele-supervision in post-disaster and low-resource settings. Curr Psychiatry Rep. 2020;22

11. Rosen CS, Morland LA, Glassman LH, Marx BP, Weaver K, Smith CA, et al. Virtual mental health care in the veterans health administration's immediate response to coronavirus disease-19. Am Psychol. 2020;

12. Pierce BS, Perrin PB, Tyler CM, McKee GB, Watson JD. The COVID-19 telepsychology revolution: a national study of pandemic-based changes in U.S. mental health care delivery. Am Psychol. 2021;76(1):14–25.
13. Mahmoud H, Vogt EL, Dahdouh R, Raymond ML. Using continuous quality improvement to design and implement a telepsychiatry program in rural Illinois. Psychiatr Serv. 2020;71(8):860–3.
14. Chan S, Li L, Torous J, Gratzer D, Yellowlees PM. Review of use of asynchronous technologies incorporated in mental health care. Curr Psychiatry Rep. 2018;20.
15. Tucker H, Lewis RB, Jose S, Lee Martin G, Over CH. Television therapy: effectiveness of closed-circuit television as a medium for therapy in treatment of the mentally ill [Internet]. Available from: https://jamanetwork.com/
16. Wittson C, Dutton R. A new tool in psychiatric education: first report from Nebraska psychiatric institute on teaching methods with closed-circuit television. Psychiatr Serv. 1956.
17. Bashshur R, Shannon G. History of telemedicine: evolution, context, and transformation. New Rochelle: Mary Ann Libert; 2009.
18. Wittson C, Affleck D, Johnson V. Two-way television in group therapy. Mental Hospitals. 1961;12(10)
19. DWYER TF. Telepsychiatry: psychiatric consultation by interactive television. Am J Psychiatr. 1973;130(8)
20. Borth D. Videophone [Internet]. Encyclopaedia Britannica, INC. 2011 [cited 2021 Jun 9]. Available from: https://www.britannica.com/technology/videophone
21. Preston J, Brown FW, Hartley B. Using telemedicine to improve health care in distant areas. Psychiatr Serv. 1992 Jan;43(1)
22. Shore J. The evolution and history of telepsychiatry and its impact on psychiatric care: current implications for psychiatrists and psychiatric organizations. Int Rev Psychiatry. 2015;27:469–75.
23. Kichloo A, Albosta M, Dettloff K, Wani F, El-Amir Z, Singh J, et al. Telemedicine, the current COVID-19 pandemic and the future: a narrative review and perspectives moving forward in the USA. Family Med Community Health. 2020;8
24. Baer L, Roderick D, Cukor P. Telepsychiatry at forty: what have we learned? 1997.
25. Krupinski EA, Antoniotti N, Bernard J. Utilization of the American telemedicine association's clinical practice guidelines. Telemedicine e-Health. 2013;19(11)
26. CMS. CMS approves first state request for 1135 medicaid waiver in Florida. Centers for Medicare & Medicaid Services. 2020.
27. Internet S, Research Maeve Duggan T. Research Associate Dana Page, Communications Manager 202.419.4372. www.pewresearch.org RECOMMENDED CITATION: Andrew Perrin, Maeve Duggan

[Internet]. Americans' Internet Access. 2000. Available from: www, pewresearch.org/internet

28. Levine S, Wein E. COVID-19: DEA and SAMHSA guidance for treating opioid use disorders via telehealth. San Fransisco: Newstex; 2020.

29. Turvey C, Coleman M, Dennison O, Drude K, Goldenson M, Hirsch P, et al. ATA practice guidelines for video-based online mental health services. Telemedicine e-Health. 2013;19:722–30.

30. American Hospital Association. Fact Sheet: Telehealth. 2019.

31. Spivak S, Spivak A, Cullen B, Meuchel J, Johnston D, Chernow R, et al. Telepsychiatry use in U.S. Mental health facilities, 2010–2017, vol. 71. Psychiatric Services; 2020. p. 121–7.

32. Barnett ML, Huskamp HA. Telemedicine for mental health in the United States: making progress, still a long way to go, vol. 71. Psychiatric Services; 2020. p. 197–8.

33. Micca P, Gibsy S, Chang C, Shukla M. Trends in health tech investments: finding the future of health. Deloitte Insights. 2021;

34. Haidous M, Tawil M, Naal H, Mahmoud H. A review of evaluation approaches for telemental health programs. Int J Psychiatry Clin Pract. 2021;25:195–205.

35. Mahmoud H, Naal H, Cerda S. Planning and implementing telepsychiatry in a community mental health setting: a case study report. Community Ment Health J. 2021;57(1):35–41.

36. Kocsis BJ, Yellowlees P. Telepsychotherapy and the therapeutic relationship: principles, advantages, and case examples. Telemedicine e-Health. 2018;24:329–34.

37. Schaffer CT, Nakrani P, Pirraglia PA. Telemental health care: a review of efficacy and interventions. Available from: https://doi.org/10.30953/tmt.v4.218

38. Hensel JM, Ellard K, Koltek M, Wilson G, Sareen J. Digital health solutions for indigenous mental well-being. Curr Psychiatry Rep. Curr Med Group LLC 1. 2019;21.

39. Mahmoud H, Vogt E. Telepsychiatry: an innovative approach to addressing the opioid crisis. J Behav Health Serv Res. 2019;46(4):680–5.

40. Mahmoud H, Sers M, Tuite J. Enhancing telemental health for rural and remote communities. Becker's Health IT; 2018.

41. Choi S, Wilcock AD, Busch AB, Huskamp HA, Uscher-Pines L, Shi Z, et al. Association of characteristics of psychiatrists with use of telemental health visits in the medicare population. JAMA Psychiatry. 2019;76(6)

42. Whaibeh E, Mahmoud H, Vogt EL. Reducing the treatment gap for LGBT mental health needs: the potential of telepsychiatry. J Behav Health Serv Res. 2020;47(3):424–31.

43. https://link.springer.com/article/10.1007/s11920-022-01352-1.

44. Zocchi M, Uscher-Pines L, Ober AJ, Kapinos KA. Costs of maintaining a high-volume telemedicine program in community health centers [Internet]. 2020. Available from: www.rand.org/giving/contribute

45. Lambert D, Gale J, Hartley D, Croll Z, Hansen A. Understanding the business case for telemental health in rural communities. J Behav Health Serv Res. 2016;43(3):366–79.
46. Shachar C, Engel J, Elwyn G. Implications for telehealth in a postpandemic future: regulatory and privacy issues. JAMA. 2020;323:2375–6.
47. Almathami HKY, Than Win K, Vlahu-Gjorgievska E. Barriers and facilitators that influence telemedicine-based, real-time, online consultation at patients' homes: systematic literature review. J. Med. Internet Res. 2020;22.
48. Mahmoud H, Vogt EL, Sers M, Fattal O, Ballout S. Overcoming barriers to larger-scale adoption of telepsychiatry. Psychiatric Ann. 2019;49:82–8.
49. Bell DJ, Self MM, Davis C, Conway F, Washburn JJ, Crepeau-Hobson F. Health service psychology education and training in the time of COVID-19: challenges and opportunities. Am Psychol. 2020;75(7)
50. Sousa J, Palimaru AI, Ober AJ, Uscher-Pines L. The case for a telemedicine coordinator: lessons learned from the sustainable models of telemedicine in the safety net initiative [Internet]. 2020. Available from: www.rand.org/giving/contribute
51. Whaibeh E, Mahmoud H, Naal H. Telemental health in the context of a pandemic: the COVID-19 experience. Curr Treatment Opt Psychiat. 2020;7(2):198–202.

The Originating Site

3

Bridget Mitchell and Hossam Mahmoud

As we saw in Chap. 2, TBH services have been successfully implemented across multiple settings, which include but are not limited to mental health centers, primary care centers, hospitals, schools, correctional facilities, federally qualified healthcare centers, First Nations tribal health centers, skilled nursing facilities, as well as patients' homes [1–4]. These physical or "brick-and-mortar" locations where patients are located at the time of receiving TBH services are called originating sites (OS) [5]. This chapter will cover OS-related aspects of TBH programs delivered to facilities with in-person staff support, including operational, clinical, and staffing considerations. Clinically unsupervised or home-based TBH services will be covered in Chap. 5.

Prior to discussing the different considerations for the OS, it is important to highlight the value of integration when delivering TBH services, especially for facility-based TBH. Integrated TBH entails delivering care into the OS, in a manner through which the teleclinician integrates into the already-existing ecosystem at the OS [6]. Both the American Psychiatric Association (APA) and the American College of Physicians (ACP) recommend inte-

B. Mitchell
Compass Health Center, Northbrook, IL, USA

H. Mahmoud (✉)
Tufts University School of Medicine, Boston, MA, USA

© The Author(s), under exclusive license to Springer Nature Switzerland AG 2022
H. Mahmoud et al. (eds.), *Essentials of Telebehavioral Health*,
https://doi.org/10.1007/978-3-030-97325-4_3

grated approaches to TBH care delivery. This includes systematic and intentional efforts by facilities and care teams to coordinate care across clinical specialties in order to address the needs of patients across the continuum of care [6, 7]. Not only does an integrated approach to TBH care mirror best practices recognized for in-person care, but it also mitigates the risk of care fragmentation [8]. This interdisciplinary approach has value, regardless of level of care, be it outpatient, residential, or inpatient settings [9].

A robust TBH program starts with robust planning around the needs of the OS and the patient population. This includes a clear understanding of the TBH services to be delivered, ICT needs, type of teleclinician, staffing resources, training needs, safety and quality protocols, regulatory processes, physical space, sustainability, and evaluation and monitoring plan [9]. Characteristics of the patient population served by the OS, such as age distribution, common BH diagnoses, substance use rates, common medical comorbidities, familiarity with technology, geographic location, and cultural characteristics, should be considered. These characteristics will guide the development of the clinical, staffing, and ICT aspects of the TBH program.

Early examination of the available resources and services within, and in the proximity of, the OS may assist you in developing appropriate workflows to support your TBH program, influence your treatment approach, and guide internal and external referrals. For example, the location and type of the OS provide substantial information on the medical resources, BHS, and psychosocial support available to the patients [10]. In addition, examining current wait-times, anticipated volume of patients, OS staffing, and program funding would guide a projection of the number of hours of services and the types of clinical services needed [5, 6].

Identifying the needs of the patient population and OS, as well as resources and ICT, will allow for planning a TBH program that meets the identified needs and mitigates anticipated barriers for successful implementation [5]. As we will see below, having standardized workflows and protocols early on are key to successful implementation, as they align the roles of the OS staff and teleclinician with the resources and technology of the OS to effectively address the needs of the patient population [5].

Geographic Location

The geographic location of the OS where patients are located is a strong factor in planning your program or practice (see Example 3.1). It has been long recognized that location [11] and place of residence are geographic social determinants of health (SDOH) that influence health needs and outcomes. This is due to convergence of SDOH, such as geographic location, socioeconomic status, food insecurity, and housing and environmental factors, affecting mental health, modifying the risk of mental illness, and impacting outcomes for individuals with mental health conditions [12, 13]. The geographic location also has cultural implications, which may shape attitudes toward the teleclinician, technology, and the use of ICT in delivering healthcare [14].

The location also reflects the community resources available for both patients and teleclinicians [5]. For example, some facilities might be located in areas with limited healthcare resources such as psychological testing, laboratory tests, imaging studies, or electrocardiograms (EKGs), to name a few. Accordingly, your TBH program should consider available ancillary services, specialized treatment options, or higher levels of care that exist locally for patients who may require them. Another example pertains to the limited Internet bandwidth in some rural areas. This may require modifications that enhance connectivity through Internet hotspots or may require minimizing OS Internet usage during TBH sessions.

In addition, the location of the OS prompts significant regulatory, financial, and cultural considerations [5], which we will discuss in detail in Chaps. 4 and 7. They include licensure requirements, reimbursement regulations, sociocultural factors, and jurisdiction-specific laws that govern the delivery of BHS.

Example 3.1 Impact of Geographic Location on Resources

The authors of this chapter oversaw the implementation of a TBH program serving a Federally Qualified Health Center (FQHC) in Michigan. The program operated across multiple different clinic sites in the Detroit area, where patients had difficulties filling prescriptions for stimulants at the local pharmacies. There had been several instances of theft of these medications at local pharmacies, so as a safety precaution, the pharmacies either stopped carrying stimulants or would only have them available in limited circumstances or small amounts, with limited medication options. The FQHC surfaced this issue to us during the implementation phase as they wanted to ensure that the teleclinician would be aware of this as they worked with patients for whom these medications may be prescribed. To minimize what otherwise would have been inefficient, and costly frequent involvement from the teleclinician in communications with the patients and pharmacies as these scripts were filled, a member of the OS staff was identified as a liaison who could offer support to patients as they obtained scripts sent by the teleclinician. While we were unable to mitigate the root cause of the issue of limited medication supplies, we were still able to align on a solution that leveraged OS site staff resources to preserve the teleclinician's time for caring for patients.

Type of Originating Sites

TBH can be delivered in clinically supervised and unsupervised OSs. Clinically supervised OSs, also known as facility-based TBH services, are those where other clinical personnel and support staff are present to provide assistance in the delivery of TBH services, before, during, or after sessions. In such OSs, on-site staff collaborate with teleclinicians and coordinate the delivery of TBH services to meet the clinical and psychosocial needs of the patient population [5]. Facility-based TBH services vary significantly by OS as every institution has its own site-specific protocols and workflows, which support the delivery of care but can create complexities as well. For instance, a correctional facility may have specific regulations and limited capacity to transport patients due to internal safety protocols, which may limit or dictate rigid time frames in which sessions can be conducted [15]. Knowledge of this specific facility nuance would ensure that patients can be scheduled appropriately and that the teleclinician with commensurate availability can be identified for the program.

Clinically unsupervised OSs, also known as home-based TBH services, include patient homes, private offices, or other private personal locations that are not healthcare facilities and usually lack the in-person support staff available at clinically supervised OS. Despite numerous advantages in expanding access to care in a manner that is convenient for patients, clinically unsupervised OSs may create challenges related to managing technology and clinical emergencies. It is important to appreciate any such challenges and plan accordingly. TBH care delivery in clinically unsupervised OSs is discussed in detail in Chap. 5. However, as an example, emergency planning and management in this context would require obtaining the phone numbers of local emergency services, family members, or significant others to be prepared to effectively assist the patient during an emergency [16].

Physical Setup

When it comes to the physical setup of the OS room to which TBH services are delivered, the general advice is that it should mimic as much as possible an in-person patient examination room in a brick-and-mortar healthcare setting. As such, the environment needs to be welcoming and relaxing with minimal distractions. While there are likely to be site-specific variations, privacy, adequate lighting, and the ability to clearly see, hear, and understand the teleclinician and patient are paramount [5]. Below are key features of the physical space of which you should be mindful.

Accessibility

While we recognize that in most public places accessibility accommodations are legal requirements, especially for health-care structures, it is important to point out that this applies to OSs for TBH services. For facility-based TBH, make sure that the allotted space is easily accessible to patients with physical limitations. If not, identify an alternative space that all patients can easily access, with minimal assistance. If that is not possible, other adaptations can be implemented to improve accessibility, such as installing a wheelchair ramp or lift if no elevator is available.

Privacy

The patient's room at the OS should be considered a "patient examination room" regardless of the intended use [9]. Ensure that the space in which the patient is sitting is private with a door that can be closed. If not, consider an alternative space or alter the space to ensure privacy. Make sure that the conversations happening inside the room cannot be overheard by other people present on site, whether they be staff members or other patients. Since this can be particularly challenging in smaller facilities with fewer resources, one low-cost option is to add a white noise machine directly outside the room in order to muffle the sound of conversations within the space. You might also consider using wall coverings or soundproofing tiles to help absorb noise and minimize sound interference.

Atmosphere

This is somewhat setting dependent, but it is important that the space be comfortable for patients [17]. Be mindful of seating arrangements in waiting rooms, as patients might be expected to wait there for an extended length of time. The same measures implemented to ensure privacy can also contribute to a more comfortable, quieter atmosphere for patients that minimizes noises, interruptions, and other distractions. Consideration should be given to the physical setup of the seating and ICT with which patients will engage to ensure that patients can comfortably sustain eye contact with the screen for an extended period of time. Ideally, the patient and teleclinician cameras should be positioned at eye level so that each person can clearly see the other's face [18].

Communication

Ensure that the teleclinician and patient can easily communicate. Echo can be a common problem in some rooms. This can be mitigated by the addition of rugs to the space or providing headphones to the patient. The space where the patient is present should be appropriately lit. Appropriately placed lighting will ensure the teleclinician can see the facial expressions and movements of the patient on screen. Depending on sources of light and time of day, window shades might need to be drawn or light sources repositioned. Make sure that the patient is not sitting directly by a window because backlighting may increase shadows and black space in the shot, which will result in low visibility for the patient. Light sources should come from above and in front of the patient.

Safety

Similar to in-person care, steps should be proactively taken to ensure the safety of patients and of on-site OS staff. We recognize that there is a wide range of safety measures that facilities may adopt, depending on location, crime rates, and history of violence and safety issues within the facility or healthcare system itself. Certain settings will dictate increased stringency on what items may be permitted in the room and what patients may bring with them to the OS. For example, correctional settings may limit items in the room to a single computer that is affixed to a table; an inpatient facility may remove any items from a room that could result in self-harm. The teleclinician must be trained on the safety protocols specific to individual OS prior to initiating TBH services.

Teleclinician

Efforts should be made to recruit a teleclinician whose qualifications, attitude, and experience match the clinical and cultural needs of the patient population [5] (Example 3.2). When possible, the OS should arrange a site visit for the teleclinician to meet the OS staff and, possibly, representatives from the patient population. In addition, cultural facilitators can be used for training the teleclinician on the local environment and culture [19]. Such cultural training has been documented to help facilitate culturally appropriate TBH services, particularly for First Nations communities (see Toolbox 3.1) [20].

Similar to in-person care, delivering TBH services requires teleclinician credentialing and privileging. Credentialing is the process of verifying and evaluating the clinician's qualifications, whereas privileging refers to the process of granting the qualified clinician authorization to deliver care and services within a particular healthcare site or system [21]. The teleclinician must be credentialed and privileged with the facility in order to deliver integrated TBH services, access the Electronic Health Record (EHR) system, electronically prescribe, and use internal ICT. In addition, the teleclinician

Toolbox 3.1 Teleclinician Quality Checklist
- Education
- Training
- Certification
- Relevant clinical experience
- ICT expertise
- Professionalism
- Flexibility
- Cultural competency

should be credentialed with payers if the facility is planning to bill insurance providers for the TBH services. Credentialing and privileging can be time consuming, so efforts to expedite them should be pursued. This could include coordinating the processes with the teleclinician and OS staff during the early planning phases of the TBH program and using electronic documents, centralized databases, and signatures when possible and legal [5, 22].

TBH programs must plan for situations in which the teleclinician is unavailable for after-hour needs and due to a planned or unplanned absence. Clear protocols should be developed and communicated to the teleclinician, OS staff, and patients to address urgent or emergent needs outside of a session. In addition, it is important to identify appropriate coverage for absences in advance. For teleclinicians who are prescribers, appropriate planning for patient prescriptions should be made in advance of any planned absences. For unplanned absences or extended planned absences, a backup clinician should be identified to address emergent patient needs and bridge prescriptions appropriately. Where there is more than one teleclinician prescriber supporting a TBH program, these teleclinicians can provide coverage in the case of absences. Or, if there are on-site prescribers, such as with hybrid TBH and in-person programs, these prescribers and the teleclinician can provide coverage for each other during absences. The OS may also opt to privilege a backup teleclinician, who does not support the TBH program full-time, but who is able to provide coverage for the primary teleclinician, if needed. Alternatively, coverage may include the patient's primary care provider (PCP) to manage psychotropic medications and bridge any gaps in prescriptions in the teleclinician's absence. If this approach is to be taken, the OS should confirm the willingness of the patients' PCPs to fulfill this role should the situation arise.

TBH programs employing teleclinicians that require collaboration or supervision, such as physician assistants or nurse practitioners, should also consider coverage needs for the primary collaborating psychiatrist. A backup collaborating or supervising psychiatrist should be identified to support the prescriber appropriately in the event that the primary collaborating psychiatrist is unavailable.

Site Staff

On-site OS staff deliver a variety of clinical and operational support, including credentialing and privileging of the teleclinicians, scheduling TBH sessions, checking patients in, taking vital signs, collecting clinical data, and assisting patients before, during, and after sessions. OS staff also play an integral role in responding to on-site psychiatric and medical emergencies, as well as technology-related disruptions. Medical assistants or nurses, in addition to clinical support, may also assist with administrative tasks, such as prior authorizations, and other roles that require clinical experience and that support care coordination or care integration. OS staff may also include clinicians such as PCPs, psychotherapists, and psychiatric prescribers, with whom the teleclinician may collaborate on patient care.

The scope and responsibilities of OS staff will vary with the size, setting, and resources of your program. The key is clearly defining responsibilities for different operational and clinical aspects, such as scheduling, vital signs, assisting patients during sessions, and administrative tasks [5]. Given the important roles the OS staff play in supporting the TBH program, it is important to get their buy-in through early involvement in planning and implementation, including training on new protocols and workflows.

A key role is that of the patient navigator, who assists the patients in navigating the TBH service experience. While responsibilities vary in scope depending on the OS, a patient navigator typically guides patients to and from the session room, ensures that the ICT necessary for patient–clinician communication are functioning, helps with technology troubleshooting, schedules follow-up appointments, and assists with managing emergencies when needed [5]. Navigators do not need specific credentials to perform such operational activities. However, depending on their experience, credentials, and training, a patient navigator may perform other roles, such as obtaining vital signs, verifying certain aspects of the patient's history, or helping with medication reconciliation [23].

The patient navigator plays a pivotal role not only by ensuring patients can effectively participate in their sessions but also by providing useful clinical information to the teleclinician. For example, the patient navigator can offer the teleclinician details about a patient's physical presentation, which may not be otherwise ascertained over the screen. These include signs of intoxication (including the smell of alcohol, cannabis, or other substances), changes in hygiene, or motor changes, such as gait, tics, or tremors, some of which may not be detectable through videoconferencing [17, 24].

For home-based TBH services, OS support staff may not be available, so administrative and clinical support tasks will likely be managed by the teleclinician or, in some cases, virtual support staff. Home-based services and teleclinician-related practice guidelines are discussed in Chap. 5.

Workflows and Protocols

If your TBH program is facility-based, there are likely already established operational workflows and clinical protocols in place. Where possible, we recommend using or adapting the existing workflows of the OS. This serves several purposes, including mitigating training burdens on staff who may be new to TBH, reducing the need to invest significant time and energy in building new workflows from scratch, and enhancing buy-in from staff who may have helped to develop the original workflows of the OS. Ensuring consistency across site-specific and TBH program workflows may also help patients be more comfortable with participating in a novel healthcare delivery method and experience. Examples of workflow components to consider include intake processes for patients, scheduling, patient check-in, vital signs, rooming patients, initiating a TBH session, prescribing, documentation, ending a TBH session, and scheduling follow-up appointments, to name a few.

If your TBH program is operationalized across different OSs within a multiple-site healthcare system, differences may exist in protocols or workflows across those sites. Examples of inter-site variations that influence protocols include differences in EHR systems or EHR availability across OSs, variations in OS staffing levels across sites, differences in Internet connectivity and bandwidth, or even differing regulatory frameworks when the OSs are located in different states. Wherever possible, a singular set of protocols or workflows across disparate sites should be established, but adjustments may still have to be made to accommodate for any differences in regulatory requirements, staff support, and patient populations. While it is possible to maintain a program with multiple sites and multiple protocols, it introduces complexity into operationalizing your program, particularly if a singular teleclinician is expected to follow these unique workflows. This would require more training for the teleclinician on the different workflows and protocols.

Based on the authors' experiences implementing TBH programs across multiple settings, a list of workflow considerations to consider is provided in Toolbox 3.2, along with recommendations for site-specific adaptations where applicable. Once workflows and protocols have been clearly established for your TBH program, we recommend documenting them in a singular reference document that is readily accessible to all stakeholders within the TBH program. You should also plan to review and adapt these workflows on a regular basis and communicate any changes to the teleclinician and OS staff, as well as the patients when applicable.

Toolbox 3.2 TBH Workflow Considerations

Program scope

- Type of services (e.g., psychotherapy, medication management, consultation).
- Number of weekly provided hours of each service.
- Weekly schedule of service availability (including whether a schedule is fixed or variable).
- Session duration for initial evaluations and follow-up appointments.
- Possible requirement for patients to engage in case management or other services offered by the OS.

Originating site

- Type of site and level of care (e.g., outpatient mental health program at a federally qualified health center; intensive outpatient program at a community mental health center).
- Location(s) where patients will participate in services.
- Staffing for the program, including key contacts for defined roles, such as patient navigator, intake or front desk staff, program manager, and information technology (IT) contact.
- Clearly defined staff responsibilities for every aspect of the program, including for scheduling patients, taking vital signs, emergency management, and technology issues.
- Processes for collecting, storing, and sharing protected health information (PHI).

Patient population

- Inclusion and exclusion criteria for participation in the TBH program.
- Age range of patients, diagnoses, acuity.
- Geographic, cultural, and linguistic considerations.

Teleclinician

- Credentials and licensure.
- Scope of practice.
- Contact information available to OS staff.

ICT

- EHR, e-prescribing software (if applicable), efax (if applicable).
- Videoconferencing platform.

Pre-session

- Intake, including relevant patient history gathered and relevant patient paperwork completed, such as informed consent, release of information (ROI).

- Policies on controlled substance prescribing, punctuality, no shows, rescheduling and cancellations.
- Scheduling, appointment reminders (including frequency and method(s) for reminders).
- Creating patient chart, collecting patient demographic and clinical history.
- Pretesting connectivity, hardware, and software.

During session

- Patient check-in, patient rooming, vitals.
- Initiating the videoconferencing session by designated OS staff.
- Prescribing, including acknowledgment of a controlled substance prescribing agreement, if applicable.
- Exiting sessions and scheduling follow-up appointments.
- Surveying patients for feedback on TBH session, teleclinician, and OS.
- Troubleshooting for technology failure, including staff members to contact and backup means of session completion.
- Crisis management, including staff members to contact.

Post-session

- Ordering laboratory and other testing, and obtaining testing results.
- Referrals to other healthcare professionals if needed.
- Procedure for refill requests between sessions.
- After-hours coverage for incoming questions, requests, and crisis calls.
- Outside of session teleclinician availability and response time for both urgent and nonurgent requests.
- Cross-coverage during teleclinician absence.

Information and Communication Technologies

All ICT programs and platforms used to deliver BHS in the United States must comply with HIPAA and HITECH requirements on the protection, storage, and sharing of protected health information (PHI) in order to ensure patient privacy and security of health information are protected. HIPAA stands for the Health Insurance Portability and Accountability Act, a federal law that regulates the protection, storage, and communication of PHI [25]. PHI refers to individually identifiable data pertaining to the health status of a person that a HIPAA-covered entity collects, creates, maintains, or transmits in the context of healthcare service delivery, payment, or operations [26]. HITECH stands for the Health Information Technology for Economic and Clinical Health Act, a federal law aimed at promoting the adoption and use of health information technology, with an emphasis on the privacy and security of health information transmitted by electronic means [27]. This means that HIPAA and HITECH compliance is required for documentation, prescribing, videoconferencing platforms, and all forms of electronic communication that may contain PHI. ICT is covered in detail in Chap. 6.

Documentation

Access to the EHR should be provided to the teleclinician if the OS utilizes an EHR system. Using an EHR system is ideal for TBH as it can facilitate secure documentation and communication of PHI between the teleclinician, staff, and other healthcare providers. While an EHR system may require upfront investments, such as the cost of licensing the software and training staff, it can increase the efficiency of documentation and eliminate the burden on OS staff to manually manage and transmit documentation, contributing to program cost-efficiency. EHR can also improve care integration and coordination by centralizing the storage and transmission of PHI among all clinicians and staff engaged in patient care [28]. A database of EHR software can be found at https://surescripts.com/network-connections/eprescribing-prescriber-software.

Some healthcare facilities continue to use paper-based charts, even for TBH service delivery. This requires downloading, printing, scanning, and, at times, mailing documents, which creates significant inefficiencies, particularly in the context of remote healthcare delivery. The manual workflow related to paper-based documentation can lead to added costs and nonclinical administrative time to the schedule of the OS staff and teleclinician. Manual workflows may also incur additional costs for equipment, such as scanners, printers, and shredders, to ensure the teleclinician can prepare, transmit, and securely manage PHI. In addition, storing paper charts requires space that can be costly or can otherwise be used for clinical or operational purposes. Finally, a lack of a centralized repository of patient information, which EHR systems can provide, may lead to care fragmentation, duplicative services, and medical errors.

If a manual documentation process must be used in your TBH program, there must be a clearly defined process for how PHI will be shared, updated, and maintained. This includes the type of information to be transmitted to the teleclinician for each patient before an appointment and the time frame within which the teleclinician must receive this information. The OS should also identify a secure method of transmitting documentation between the site and the teleclinician, and the teleclinician should have a defined process for disposing of any redundant copies of PHI. The OS should ensure that all documents transmitted are legible and that any documents transmitted that incorporate information entered by other clinicians or support staff are updated before sending. For example, if a Medication Administration Record (MAR) is part of the record for a patient, the OS should ensure that all medications administered or prescribed to a patient, including those prescribed by clinicians outside of the TBH program, are included in the documentation. In addition, because manually updating and transmitting documentation requires more time, this should be appropriately accounted for in the schedule of the teleclinician to ensure they have adequate time to see patients and accurately document visits.

Regardless of whether the TBH program uses an EHR system or paper documentation, templates for documenting initial evaluations, progress notes, or therapy notes should be identified to capture the necessary clinical, demographic, and location information associated with the TBH encounter. While templates vary, their use can support quality and efficiency of clinical documentation [29, 30]. In some instances, an OS may be new to BHS altogether and may not have templates. In this case, the teleclinician should work with the OS to ensure appropriate templates are developed. If the OS has current templates for BHS, the teleclinician should familiarize themselves with them and discuss any possible adjustments to meet the documentation needs of the TBH program. The APA provides guidance on the components of clinical documentation in TBH. This can be accessed at https://www.psychiatry.org/psychiatrists/practice/telepsychiatry/toolkit/clinical-documentation.

Prescribing

If your TBH program will include medication management, a method or process for remote prescribing must be identified. Similar to our recommendations on documentation, electronic prescribing (or e-prescribing) is considered optimal. e-Prescribing is the transmission of medication prescriptions directly to the pharmacy using a stand-alone software or one that is part of an EHR software [31]. e-Prescribing allows for medications to be sent more efficiently and potentially decreases errors [31]. In addition, e-prescribing minimizes the risk of lost or delayed prescriptions and, in the case of TBH, decreases the burden on the patient, who otherwise would have to wait for a mailed prescription that they then have to take to the pharmacy themselves. Like documentation, paper prescriptions require additional work on the part of the teleclinician, such as physically traveling to a post office or other shipping store to mail prescriptions to the facility or to the patient's home.

Some states and pharmacy chains require e-prescribing for all medications [31]. In addition, Electronic Prescribing of Controlled Substances (EPCS) is now allowed in all US states and the District of Columbia. Further information on EPCS can be found at the Drug Enforcement Administration website https://www.deadiversion.usdoj.gov/ecomm/e_rx/thirdparty.htm. The MD Toolbox website provides an interactive map of states that have laws mandating e-prescribing. A database of e-prescribing software can be found at https://surescripts.com/network-connections/eprescribing-prescriber-software.

An e-prescribing software that is integrated into the EHR is preferred for care integration. The OS should verify whether e-prescribing functionality is available within the EHR; otherwise, a separate e-prescribing software can be licensed. While licensing e-prescribing software may have added costs, such costs should be weighed against the drawbacks of paper prescriptions, such as mailing costs, associated inefficiencies, and the risk of delayed treatment or lost prescriptions.

Regardless of whether e-prescribing or paper scripts are used, a backup process should be identified in the event of a technology failure or if the teleclinician is unable to mail prescriptions. The OS and teleclinician should identify a workflow for ensuring patients receive their prescriptions in a timely fashion to avoid treatment disruption. This may include having other clinicians in the TBH program or at the OS issue interim prescriptions; having the patient's PCP prescribe the medications; or having the teleclinician call in prescriptions to the pharmacy if federal and state regulations allow. As backup prescribing methods could be time consuming, the OS should provide the teleclinician with all the pertinent information to facilitate these calls and may need to alter the teleclinician's schedule to accommodate the process.

Facility-based TBH programs should adhere to the in-person practices of the OS. For example, some OSs may have formularies, which limit which medications a teleclinician may prescribe. If this is the case, the formulary and any possible exceptions should be provided to the teleclinician and incorporated into their training. In addition, transparent discussions between the OS and teleclinician about prescribing philosophies prior to launching services are critical as misalignment on such issues may affect the provision of patient care (see Example 3.2). For example, an OS and teleclinician may have divergent prescribing philosophies for certain controlled substances, or a teleclinician may decline to prescribe certain medications for patients who use recreational substances, or an OS may have a no-controlled-substance prescribing policy.

Example 3.2 Alignment of Prescribing Philosophies and Patient Needs
Alignment between the prescribing philosophies of the teleclinician and the OS site is paramount and should be one of the topics discussed in detail prior to implementing a TBH program. The legalization of recreational and medicinal cannabis use across several US jurisdictions may result in more patients reporting cannabis use. Some prescribing teleclinicians may decline to prescribe controlled substances to these patients, even if OS support staff or other prescribing clinicians at the OS are comfortable with this practice. The authors of this chapter experienced a misalignment of these prescribing philosophies when working with a rural healthcare system in Illinois. Many patients served by that system reported using cannabis, and the expectation of the OS staff was that some of these patients could still be prescribed certain controlled substances. The teleclinician, on the other hand, was strongly opposed to prescribing controlled substances for any patients who reported using cannabis. However, prior to deployment of services, this particular prescribing approach had not been discussed with the teleclinician, who was otherwise considered a good fit for the needs of this program and held the appropriate licensure, training, and credentials required to serve the population.

Ultimately, the OS determined that a clinician with a pre-scribing philosophy aligned with theirs would be a better fit for their patients, and a search for a new teleclinician was initiated. While the new teleclinician was able to meet the needs of some patients in a manner that the OS support staff felt was more beneficial, the transition required lengthy privileging and credentialing processes for the new telecli-nician. Additionally, care transition was challenging for some patients who had developed a positive rapport with the original teleclinician only to reestablish care with another teleclinician.

Testing

Like in-person care, TBH services may require ordering tests as part of a workup to rule out organic causes of BH symptoms for medical clearance prior to choosing a medication, monitoring medication levels, or assessing adherence to treatment. Examples of such testing include thyroid panel, urine drug screen, EKG, brain imaging, and metabolic panel, to name a few. Like documentation and prescribing, a process for ordering tests should be defined prior to launching TBH services. Where possible, the process used by the OS should be leveraged for the TBH program. Increasingly, more EHRs have functionality that allows remote ordering of tests to a variety of laboratories and testing centers. Remember that the protocol and processes for notifying the tele-clinician and the patient of testing results, including critical results, should also be identified.

Crisis Management

While managing BH and medical emergencies can be challenging regardless of setting, a remotely located patient requires adjust-ments to safety and emergency protocols in sessions. If a teleclinician identifies that a patient is experiencing a BH or medical emergency during a facility-based TBH session, such as risk of harm to themselves or others, or concerning medical symptoms, the teleclinician should follow the emergency protocol outlined by the OS to ensure rapid crisis response. This emergency protocol must be clearly documented and regularly reviewed and updated as needed [5]. A crisis management plan should include

- The crisis protocols of the OS, including their standard processes for managing patients in emergency situations [6, 32].
- The OS staff point person(s) to be contacted for crisis management, as well as their contact information.
- The method by which the teleclinician will contact this point person.

While BH clinicians are usually trained in crisis management and de-escalation techniques, crisis management protocols specific to the OS should be discussed during the teleclinician's onboarding. The OS should also ensure that all staff supporting the TBH program are trained in crisis management and de-escalation techniques.

If the OS does not have a crisis management protocol, the teleclinician and OS can collaborate to develop crisis management procedures that may include identifying local healthcare facilities, emergency departments (EDs), and local emergency service phone numbers, as well as having contact information and ROI for the patient's social supports [32].

After-Hours Coverage

As with in-person services, the policies for addressing after-hours questions or concerns related to TBH services should be clearly defined and communicated to the patients, OS staff and the teleclinician [33]. These may include policies on methods of communication and expectations for response time by the teleclinician for after-hours queries.

Depending on the staffing resources, there are variations in how facilities handle crisis calls after hours. This may involve having OS staff on call, outsourcing crisis management, or directing to local or national crisis hotlines. Psychiatric emergencies that require safety management should be directed to an appropriate in-person resource, including a local ED or community crisis intervention service. After-hours crisis calls must be documented and communicated to the teleclinician.

Training

OS staff and teleclinician should receive training on TBH-specific workflows and protocols, including the elements described throughout this chapter. The training checklist includes [5]

- ICT, software, hardware, troubleshooting
- EHR, e-prescribing, e-faxing, ordering tests
- Facility policies and procedures that impact BHS delivery and practices
- Process for managing requests outside of the teleclinician's regularly scheduled hours
- Introductions to all team members supporting the TBH program, with clear roles and responsibilities
- Cultural training
- Crisis management protocols
- HIPAA compliance
- Online security

References

1. Yellowlees P, Burke MM, Marks SL, Hilty DM, Shore JH. Emergency telepsychiatry. J Telemed Telecare. 2008;14(6).
2. Nelson E-L, Cain S, Sharp S. Considerations for conducting telemental health with children and adolescents. Child Adolesc Psychiatr Clin N Am. 2017;26(1).

3. Leonard S. The development and evaluation of a telepsychiatry service for prisoners. J Psychiatr Ment Health Nurs. 2004;11(4).
4. Spivak S, Spivak A, Cullen B, Meuchel J, Johnston D, Chernow R, et al. Telepsychiatry use in U.S. Mental health facilities, 2010–2017. Psychiatric Services. 2020;71:121–7.
5. Mahmoud H, Whaibeh E, Mitchel B. Ensuring successful telepsychiatry program implementation: critical components and considerations Curr Treatment Opt Psychiat. 2020.
6. Shore JH, Yellowlees P, Caudill R, Johnston B, Turvey C, Mishkind M, et al. Best practices in videoconferencing-based telemental health April 2018. Telemedicine e-Health. 2018;24(11):827–32.
7. Daniel H, Sulmasy LS, Delong DM, Beachy MW, Bornstein SS, Bush JF, et al. Policy recommendations to guide the use of telemedicine in primary care settings: an American College of Physicians position paper. Ann Intern Med. 2015;163(10):787–9.
8. Ray Dorsey E, Topol EJ. State of telehealth. N Engl J Med. 2016;375(2):154–61.
9. APA. APA and ATA release new telemental health guide. American Psychiatric Association; 2018.
10. Mahmoud H, Whaibeh E, Mitchell B. Ensuring successful telepsychiatry program implementation: critical components and considerations. Curr Treatment Opt Psychiat. 2020;7(2):186–97.
11. WHO. Social determinants of mental health. Geneva; 2014.
12. Shim RS, Compton MT. The social determinants of mental health: psychiatrists' roles in addressing discrimination and food insecurity. Focus. 2020;18(1):25–30.
13. Leonard T, Hughes AE, Donegan C, Santillan A, Pruitt SL. Overlapping geographic clusters of food security and health: where do social determinants and health outcomes converge in the U.S? SSM – Population Health. 2018;(5):160–70.
14. Shore JH, Savin D, Novins D, Manson SM. Cultural aspects of telepsychiatry. J Telemed Telecare. 2006;12(3):116–21.
15. Deslich S. Telepsychiatry in correctional facilities: using technology to improve access and decrease costs of mental health care in underserved populations. Perm J. 2013;17(3).
16. Norris D, Bursztajn H, Gutheil T, Brodsky A. Telepsychiatry: practical pointers and potential pitfalls. Psychiatric Times. 2021.
17. Shore JH. Telepsychiatry: videoconferencing in the delivery of psychiatric care. Am J Psychiatr. 2013;170(3):256–62.
18. Shore JH, Yellowlees P, Caudill R, Johnston B, Turvey C, Mishkind M, et al. Best practices in videoconferencing-based telemental health. WRITING COMMITTEE; 2018.
19. Mishkind MC. Establishing telemental health services from conceptualization to powering up. Psychiatr Clin N Am. 2019;42(4).

20. Kruse CS, Bouffard S, Dougherty M, Parro JS. Telemedicine use in rural native American communities in the era of the ACA: a systematic literature review. J Med Syst

21. JCA. Ambulatory Care Program: The Who, What, When and Where's of Credentialing and Privileging.

22. Lokken TG, Blegen RN, Hoff MD, Demaerschalk BM. Overview for implementation of telemedicine services in a large integrated multispecialty health care system. Telemedicine e-Health. 2019;00(00):1–6.

23. Cash C. Telepsychiatry and risk management. Innovations in clinical Neuroscience. 2011;8(9).

24. Mahmoud H, Vogt EL, Sers M, Fattal O, Ballout S. Overcoming barriers to larger-scale adoption of telepsychiatry. Psychiatr Ann. 2019;49(2):82–8.

25. CDC. Health Insurance Portability and Accountability Act of 1996 (HIPAA). Center for Disease Control and Prevention; 2018.

26. HIPAA. What is considered protected health information under HIPAA. HIPAA J. 2021.

27. HHS. HITECH Act Enforcement Interim Final Rule. U.S Department of Health & Human Services. 2017.

28. Improve care coordination: the need for better, improved care coordination. Health IT. 2017.

29. Mehta R, Radhakrishnan N, Warring C, Jain A, Fuentes J, Dolganiuc A, et al. The use of evidence-based, problem-oriented templates as a clinical decision support in an inpatient electronic health record system. Appl Clin Informatics. 2016;07(03).

30. Bajgier J, Bender J, Ries R. Use of templates for clinical documentation in psychiatric evaluations—beneficial or counterproductive for residents in training? Int J Psychiatry Med. 2012;43(1).

31. APA. E-prescribing (eRx). American Psychiatric Association; 2021.

32. ATA. Practice guidelines for video-based online mental health services; 2013.

33. ATA. Core Operational Guidelines for Telehealth Services Involving Provider-Patient Interactions.

The Patient Population

4

Hossam Mahmoud, Emile Whaibeh,
and Fayth Dickenson

Patient Population

TBH has been demonstrated to be effective and feasible with many patient populations for a wide range of diagnoses and across different healthcare settings [1–3]. According to the APA and ATA, no absolute patient contraindications exist for assessing or treating patients through TBH [4]. Rather, in order to most effectively tailor your practice, you must understand and consider the needs of the patients to whom you will deliver BHS [5]. In addition to the information covered in the previous chapter on the sociocultural, environmental, and geographic landscape of the OS, additional patient-specific considerations should be factored into the design of your practice. These include the patient population's demographics, common diagnoses, payer composition, linguistic considerations, cultural specificities, attitudes toward TBH [5], clinical resources available to the patients, technological

H. Mahmoud
Tufts University School of Medicine, Boston, MA, USA

E. Whaibeh (✉)
Department of Public Health, Faculty of Health Sciences, University of Balamand (UOB), Beirut, Lebanon

F. Dickenson
Behavioral Health, Beacon Health Options, Boston, MA, USA

© The Author(s), under exclusive license to Springer Nature Switzerland AG 2022
H. Mahmoud et al. (eds.), *Essentials of Telebehavioral Health*,
https://doi.org/10.1007/978-3-030-97325-4_4

resources, and common barriers to accessing care [5]. What follows is a list of data points that should be gathered as part of assessing whether a patient population can be well served by a particular teleclinician or a particular TBH program:

- Demographic information: Age range and mean age of the population. Linguistic needs, racial/ethnic composition, and cultural considerations.
- Clinical information: Common BH diagnoses, common medical comorbidities, and historical rates of controlled substance prescribing needs.
- Common risk and protective factors, such as rates of substance use in the community, specific community or environmental stressors, and types of community support systems available. This also includes other SDOH, such as socioeconomic status, food insecurity, and housing factors.
- Healthcare resources available within the community: Proximity to other healthcare facilities, including urgent care centers and EDs, availability of specialized care centers, and availability of laboratories and imaging centers. Payer mix can also fall under this category as it may determine access to certain services.
- Perceptions of TBH: Perceptions among the patient population of technology use in healthcare, willingness to receive care via TBH, and previous experiences with TBH within the OS. While ideally a formal survey can be conducted to determine attitudes toward TBH, when such a survey is not feasible, anecdotal feedback from patients can be solicited by OS staff.
- The OS clinical and support staff, who can support and co-manage treatment, to address the patient population needs; it is important to ensure the alignment of the teleclinician and the OS staff on the workflows and protocols for serving the patient population.

This information will assist you in developing and implementing your TBH program, so that the OS staff and teleclinician can meet patient needs. Considerations include relevant training for teleclinicians and support staff, patient engagement approaches, crisis management protocols, ICT needs, and required operational, regulatory, and clinical processes. Such OS and teleclinician considerations are discussed in detail, with examples, in Chaps. 3 and 5. This chapter discusses different patient populations to outline both the wide applicability of TBH and patient considerations when planning your TBH program.

Child and Adolescent Populations

BH conditions are highly prevalent among US children and adolescents, with 1 in 6 of those aged between 6 and 17 years having a treatable condition such as depression, anxiety, or ADHD [6]. Despite that, many children and adolescents who need BHS either do not receive treatment, receive treatment intermittently, or receive care from clinicians who may lack the necessary specialty training for this patient population [7]. Moreover, the COVID-19 pandemic was increasingly disruptive to the lives of many families, communities, and systems of care, and exacerbated existing BH problems specifically among children and adolescents, with higher rates of anxiety, depression, and PTSD reported within that group [8]. This indicates that the BH treatment needs of this patient population are likely to continue to grow.

TBH has the potential to reduce disparities in access to BHS while simultaneously improving the quality of care that children and adolescents receive [9]. First, it is well-suited for children and adolescents, who are sometimes described as "digital natives," because they have higher levels of comfort with and exposure to ICT [7, 10]. Second, given the shortage of clinicians who specialize in treating children and adolescents, TBH services have been integral in getting care to these populations, supporting higher quality and more age-appropriate approaches to care [11]. Third, TBH reduces the time spent away from a guardian's work or a patient's school, decreases absenteeism, and cuts down the costs associated with commuting to and from in-person appointments [7]. Fourth, because TBH sessions could be delivered in settings that the child or adolescent is already familiar with, such as their home or school, the stress associated with being in new settings and the fear of stigma is reduced [7]. Finally, a unique advantage that TBH offers, especially home-based TBH, is that it makes it possible for both patients and guardians to engage in behavioral change interventions within their lived environment, and offers the possibility of receiving additional support from multiple family members or guardians than would be logistically possible in an in-person clinical setting [10].

While TBH for children and adolescents follows similar guidelines to those for adult populations, there are certain clinical considerations that should be taken into account such as the patient's developmental stage and associated language capability, cognitive capacity, and motor functioning [4]. There are also regulatory variations among different jurisdictions that pertain to the age of consent, whereby minors may consent to BHS without the requirement of a guardian or parent's consent [12]. For example, a study from 2016 reviewed US state laws on adolescent decision-making. That review found that state laws support minors' right to access SUD treatment without needing parental consent and at a younger age compared to mental health treatment, with significant variations across states and treatment settings [12]. Finally, while guardian, parent, or other family member involvement in BH treatment is typical, having a telehealth navigator present during or around facility-based TBH sessions may affect the treatment dynamic. The presence of a telehealth navigator may raise concerns about confidentiality and privacy, as well as information sharing [4]. Therefore, it is important to proactively explain the role of the telehealth navigator and discuss any concerns the child, adolescent, or guardian may have about privacy and confidentiality.

Geriatric Populations

Factors limiting access to care specifically for geriatric patient populations include specialized clinician shortage, transportation issues, and restricted physical mobility affecting their ability to travel to appointments. Thus, TBH is particularly advantageous for geriatric patients with decreased mobility, in need of transportation assistance, or living with cognitive impairment or other chronic health conditions. While TBH for the geriatric population has largely been applied in nursing homes and inpatient settings, it can also be a crucial adjunct for psychiatric consultations in the care of older adults in the community, specifically in rural and remote areas [13].

Studies support the feasibility, acceptability, and satisfaction with TBH services by geriatric patients and their caregivers, both of whom benefit from its added convenience. In addition, the literature demonstrates the validity of using TBH for cognitive and neuropsychological testing while recognizing some challenges associated with certain testing components that include tasks, such as drawing a clock [4]. Communication issues are among the highest noted challenges for both patients and clinicians in this scenario resulting from possible sensorineural deficits, difficulty utilizing ICT, or potential technology malfunctions. Clinicians found the need to repeat questions disruptive, and patient feedback commonly included complaints about unclear audio [14].

More studies are needed to guide the development of TBH programs for older adults, and particularly to take into consideration age-related changes in hearing, vision, and attention. That said, TBH has proven to be impactful in decreasing ED utilization and hospital admissions, as well as improving depressive symptoms and cognitive functioning among geriatric patients. The following is a list of considerations when delivering TBH services to this patient population:

- Due to higher rates of comorbidities among older adults, all aspects of behavioral and medical health needs should be monitored and addressed. This requires collaboration and care integration with a potentially wide array of healthcare professionals involved in the patient's care.
- The patient's living situation should be assessed for both social supports and barriers that may contribute to, or interfere with, the ability to access and maintain treatment. Family members and caregivers should be involved when clinically appropriate and with patient permission. As with many home-based

services, privacy issues may arise, but that setting may also allow for additional technical assistance and family or caregiver input if needed [14].

- Consideration should be given to any prior experience the patient may have had with TBH or traditional BHS, positive or negative [14]. In many circumstances, the teleclinician can process that experience with the patient and build on it to improve therapeutic alliance and treatment plan adherence.
- Auditory enhancements may help with the user experience, though more robust research is needed on the use of geriatric-specific devices, requiring individual patient consideration [14]. Some examples include adjusting volume settings, offering closed on-screen captioning options with enhanced text size, and using headphone sets or earphones.
- Prior to appointments, providing written instructions for using ICT that include concise language, a larger font size, or screenshots of each step of the process can be helpful.

Rural Populations

Teleclinicians should familiarize themselves with the sociocultural and geographic landscape of their patient populations [15]. This includes familiarizing oneself with the healthcare services and resources available in a particular region, as well as historical and ongoing barriers to care [15]. This is of particular significance for rural populations, which face a combination of BH challenges, including increased psychosocial and geographical stressors, coupled with significant access challenges to BHS. For example, some rural populations face higher levels of stress compared to urban areas, including higher levels of unemployment and poverty, as well as elevated vulnerability to natural disasters and accidents [16]. In addition, the opioid epidemic and overdose-related deaths have particularly affected rural communities [17]. On the other hand, many barriers to BH treatment exist, with elevated rates of stigma, limited healthcare infrastructure, fewer psychosocial services, and a shortage of qualified BH clinicians [17]. It continues to be difficult to recruit and retain BH professionals in rural areas, leaving a large percentage of the rural population of the United States with very limited access to BHS [15]. These barriers have historically led to a phenomenon referred to by some as "greyhound therapy," whereby rural residents have to travel to urban areas to access BHS, leading to significant travel costs and burdens, as well as lost work hours. TBH can immensely benefit underserved rural populations by mitigating the effects of the shortage of BH professionals in rural areas, minimizing travel time and costs, and bypassing stigma [15].

LGBTQ Communities

Lesbian, Gay, Bisexual, Transgender, and Queer or Questioning (LGBTQ) individuals are at higher risk than their non-LGBTQ counterparts of developing BH conditions. This does not inherently result from their sexual or gender identities, but rather, as demonstrated by the minority stress model, it is associated with the discrimination, violence, and civil and human rights violations which they experience. At the same time, LGBTQ individuals encounter barriers to accessing care, ranging from denial of treatment altogether to difficulties finding LGBTQ-affirming clinicians. At the individual level, LGBTQ individuals face a double stigma, one associated with BH conditions and the other with their LGBTQ minority status. At the clinician level, LGBTQ individuals continue to face discriminatory attitudes and behaviors from some clinicians in the context of a shortage of clinicians trained in the care of LGBTQ individuals. At a systemic level, LGBTQ individuals face institutional discrimination, as well as anti-LGBTQ laws, some of which allow clinicians to refuse care for LGBTQ patients or prevent clinicians from providing LGBTQ appropriate care [18, 19].

TBH offers opportunities for clinicians to deliver BH services that are appropriate for LGBTQ individuals, bypassing many of the aforementioned barriers. At the individual level, TBH bypasses stigma and has been associated with enhancing the ease of provider-patient communication for LGBTQ patients when compared to in-person care. At the clinician level, TBH provides LGBTQ patients expanded opportunities to receive care from culturally appropriate teleclinicians, regardless of location. At the systemic level, TBH reduces or eliminates the time and burden of travel to receive affirming care, especially when personal safety is an issue during travel [18].

Populations with Substance Use Disorders

Patients with SUD face many challenges accessing care, particularly in rural areas, where there are limited treatment resources, limited treatment facilities, and a shortage of addiction specialists [18]. This is compounded by stigma, which may discourage patients with SUD from seeking treatment [18]. These barriers are particularly challenging because treatment for SUD usually requires structured programs that incorporate psychosocial services and pharmacotherapy and that include regular follow-up [20].

TBH is effective in treating a variety of SUDs [18, 21], including the delivery of medication-assisted treatment (MAT) and other therapeutic modalities [18, 21–23]. MAT is defined as the use of medications, alongside psychotherapy, to treat SUDs including opioid use disorders (OUDs). Medications prescribed will depend on the SUD being treated and can include disulfiram, acamprosate, naltrexone, buprenorphine, and naloxone [24].

In addition to being convenient and eliminating the need to travel for services, TBH can bypass the stigma barrier by making treatment more "low profile" and thereby enhancing patients' privacy [3]. This aspect appears to be particularly helpful in rural communities [3], where stigma associated with BHS and especially SUDs tends to be more pervasive compared to more urban settings. TBH-delivered MAT was further supported by the Drug Enforcement Agency's position supporting the prescribing of buprenorphine remotely in accordance with the Ryan Haight Act [25]. However, given the variations in regulations by jurisdictions, teleclinicians must familiarize themselves with local regulations on prescribing controlled substances, including buprenorphine [4].

Patients with Communication Needs

As in the case of in-person care, TBH services can be modified to serve patients with particular communication needs. These may include challenges with auditory, visual, and speech communication, or with linguistic differences.

If the patients, teleclinicians, or OS staff speak different languages, language interpreters would be needed. Interpreters could be located at the OS or could join via videoconferencing or audio calls to facilitate sessions. Keep in mind that the use of "informal" interpreters, such as the telehealth navigator, family members, or others without formal training as interpreters, may lead to miscommunication of clinical complaints, de-emphasizing certain pieces of information, or causing misunderstanding of the clinical narrative or of cultural metaphors [26].

Sign language for patients with hearing impairment can work well with videoconferencing [27] since sign language interpreters may be located at the OS or can join via videoconferencing. We recommend three approaches to accommodate patients with hearing impairment that can also be used simultaneously when possible or needed [28]:

- Direct participation of interpreters remotely using the same platform.
- Direct captioning of the session by qualified captioners, using the same platform. This is also referred to as Communication Access Real-time Translation (CART).
- Using remote captioning or interpreting on a separate screen, platform, or device.

Finally, TBH may offer particular advantages for patients with impaired vision by eliminating the need for travel. Because patients with visual impairment may not be able to interpret non-verbal cues, the teleclinician and OS staff should communicate clearly, solicit regular patient feedback, and provide assistance with technology, when specialized software or hardware is unavailable. Examples of aids for patients with impaired vision may include providing information and instructions in Braille, using large print, or utilizing ICT that offers screen-reading capabilities. Other options include providing information and instructions through a qualified reader or in the form of an audio recording [29].

Informed Consent and Patient Information

As with in-person care, patients accessing treatment through TBH must be provided with information on patient rights and responsibilities, type of service, billing practices, and scheduling process (see Toolbox 4.1).

The consent process should incorporate the circumstances that may lead to discontinuation of TBH services and referral to in-person treatment, in cases where the patient cannot be treated remotely [30]. Patients must also be informed of policies on communication, including boundaries pertaining to communication modality with the teleclinician during and between appointments, expected response times, mandated reporting, confidentiality, and the type of information appropriate to be communicated over different platforms [4, 30]. In addition, patients must be informed of protocols for crisis management, including BH emergencies, medical emergencies, and technological failure [4].

Toolbox 4.1 Key Points Under a TBH Service Informed Consent and Patient Information

Definition of TBH

- Benefits of TBH services
  - Increased access, decrease wait-times, and convenience
- Risks
  - Possible technological failure (hardware, software, Internet connectivity), leading to service interruptions during sessions, suboptimal communication, or limited video resolution
  - Protocol in case of technological failure, usually switching to phone
  - Possibility that service interruption due to technological failure may lead to cancellation, rescheduling, delays in treatment
- Information on OS staff roles and responsibilities, after-hour and inter-appointment availability, crisis management, and e-prescribing
- Possible situations that may lead to service termination

Patient rights

- Federal and jurisdiction-specific laws and regulations govern the delivery of BHS, including those that apply to TBH services.
- Confidentiality and privacy are regulated and protected with TBH, as with in-person care
- Protected health information (PHI) will be stored and communicated in a secure, encrypted, and HIPAA-compliant manner (HIPAA Notice of Privacy Practices.)
- TBH sessions will not be recorded without written patient authorization.
- Only individuals authorized by both patient and teleclinician will be allowed to be present on either end during TBH sessions.

Patient responsibilities

- TBH sessions will not be recorded without written tele-clinician authorization.
- Only individuals authorized by both patient and teleclinician will be allowed to be present on either end during TBH session.
- OS policies for in-person care also apply to TBH (for home-based services, the teleclinician's or facility's policies apply.)
- The patient is expected to adhere to policies, including on scheduling, cancellation, rescheduling, and missed appointment policies.
- The patient is expected to adhere to other communicated policies that may be site specific or teleclinician specific

Patient consent

- Section on having read and understood the above information
- Section on having had answers to questions on the above sections answered
- Section on medication prescribing
- Signature section

Referring Patients to In-person BHS

While most patients can be served using TBH, some patients may need to be referred to in-person care. Specifically in the absence of in-person staff support, the APA recommends that the following consideration be incorporated as a teleclinician assesses patient appropriateness for TBH services [4]:

- ICT capabilities: ability to utilize ICT, including videoconferencing software and hardware

- Location: geographic location and proximity to medical facilities
- BH needs, cognitive capacity, substance use, history of violence, history of self-harm, and patient's support system
- Medical needs: comorbid medical conditions and possible need for physical examination

Note that the above scenarios typically apply to outpatient TBH; however, since COVID-19, there has been an increase in the delivery of TBH services into higher levels of care [31], including IOP, PHP, and residential and inpatient settings. Therefore, assessing patient appropriateness should take into consideration the needs of the patient, clinical setting, support staff, and intensity of services. Resources available to support the patient, at the OS or through collaboration with other treatment teams, should also be considered, along with the involvement of family members and other support systems available to the patient.

Examples of scenarios that may lead to referring patients to in-person care [30]:

- Imminent risk of harm to self or others
- Active self-harm behaviors or active suicidal ideations
- Severe psychosis or disorientation that impairs a patient's ability to engage with services remotely
- History of violence
- History of limited engagement with treatment
- Frequent ED utilization
- Frequent utilization of higher clinical levels of care, such as inpatient hospitalization, residential programs, PHP, or IOP
- Connectivity issues that compromise the ability to engage in sessions
- Inability to use ICT for BHS
- Unwillingness to engage in BHS through ICT
- Patient preference
- Limited progress in treatment through TBH

References

1. Mahmoud H, Vogt EL, Sers M, Fattal O, Ballout S. Overcoming barriers to larger-scale adoption of telepsychiatry. Psychiatr Ann. 2019;49(2):82–8.
2. Hensel JM, Ellard K, Koltek M, Wilson G, Sareen J. Digital health solutions for indigenous mental well-being. Curr Psychiatry Rep. 2019;21(8).
3. Mahmoud H, Vogt E. Telepsychiatry: an innovative approach to addressing the opioid crisis. J Behav Health Serv Res. 2019;46(4):680–5.
4. Shore JH, Yellowlees P, Caudill R, Johnston B, Turvey C, Mishkind M, et al. Best practices in videoconferencing-based telemental health. WRITING COMMITTEE; 2018.
5. Mahmoud H, Whaibeh E, Mitchel B. Ensuring successful telepsychiatry program implementation: critical components and considerations Curr Treatment Opt Psychiat. 2020.
6. Whitney D, Peterson M. US National and State-Level Prevalence of Mental Health Disorders and Disparities of Mental Health Care Use in Children. 2019;173(4):389–91.
7. Nelson E-L, Cain S, Sharp S. Considerations for conducting telemental health with children and adolescents. Child Adolesc Psychiatr Clin N Am. 2017;26(1).
8. Ros-De Marize R, Chung P, Stewart R. Pediatric behavioral telehealth in the age of COVID-19: brief evidence review and practice considerations. Curr Prob Pediatric Adolescent Health Care. 2021;51(1).
9. Gloff NE, LeNoue SR, Novins DK, Myers K. Telemental health for children and adolescents. Int Rev Psychiat. 2015;27(6).
10. Monzon AD, Zhang E, Marker AM, Nelson E-L. Overview of child tele-behavioral interventions using real-time videoconferencing. In: Telemedicine, telehealth and telepresence. Cham: Springer International Publishing; 2021.
11. Kramer GM, Luxton DD. Telemental health for children and adolescents: an overview of legal, regulatory, and risk management issues. J Child Adolesc Psychopharmacol. 2016;26(3).
12. Kerwin ME, Kirby KC, Speziali D, Duggan M, Mellitz C, Versek B, et al. What can parents do? A review of state laws regarding decision making for adolescent drug abuse and mental health treatment. J Child Adolesc Subst Abuse. 2015;24(3).
13. Dham P, Gupta N, Alexander J, Black W, Rajji T, Skinner E. Community based telepsychiatry service for older adults residing in a rural and remote region- utilization pattern and satisfaction among stakeholders. BMC Psychiat. 2018;18(1).
14. Harerimana B, Forchuk C, O'Regan T. The use of technology for mental healthcare delivery among older adults with depressive symptoms: a systematic literature review. Int J Ment Health Nurs. 2019;28(3).

15. Mahmoud H, Sers M, Tuite J. Enhancing telemental health for rural and remote communities. Becker's Health IT. 2018.
16. Simms DC, Gibson K, O'Donnell S. To use or not to use: clinicians' perceptions of telemental health. Can Psychol. 2011;52(1).
17. Lister JJ, Weaver A, Ellis JD, Himle JA, Ledgerwood DM. A systematic review of rural-specific barriers to medication treatment for opioid use disorder in the United States. Am J Drug Alcohol Abuse. 2020;46(3).
18. Whaibeh E, Mahmoud H, Vogt EL. Reducing the treatment gap for LGBT mental health needs: the potential of telepsychiatry. J Behav Health Serv Res. 2020;47(3):424–31.
19. Ronan W. BREAKING: 2021 becomes record year for anti-transgender legislation. Human Rights Campaign; 2021.
20. WHO. Guidelines for the psychosocially-assisted pharmacological treatment of opioid dependence. Geneva; 2009.
21. Kruse CS, Lee K, Watson JB, Lobo LG, Stoppelmoor AG, Oyibo SE. Measures of effectiveness, efficiency, and quality of telemedicine in the management of alcohol abuse, addiction, and rehabilitation: systematic review. J Med Internet Res. 2020;22(1).
22. Blalock D, Calhoun PS, Crowley MJ, Dedert EA. Telehealth treatment for alcohol misuse: reviewing telehealth approaches to increase engagement and reduce risk of alcohol-related hypertension. Curr Hypertension Rep. 2019;21(8).
23. Mahmoud H, Naal H, Whaibeh E, Smith A. Telehealth-Based Delivery of Medication-Assisted Treatment for Opioid Use Disorder: a Critical Review of Recent Developments. Curr Psychiatry Rep. https://www.samhsa.gov/medication-assisted-treatment.
24. U.S Food and Drug Administration. Information about medication-assisted treatment (MAT); 2019.
25. Telemedicine and prescribing buprenorphine for the treatment of opioid use disorder. U.S Department of Health and Human Services. 2018.
26. Hilty DM, Gentry MT, McKean AJ, Cowan KE, Lim RF, Lu FG. Telehealth for rural diverse populations: telebehavioral and cultural competencies, clinical outcomes and administrative approaches. mHealth. 2020;6.
27. Hilty DM, Ferrer DC, Parish MB, Johnston B, Callahan EJ, Yellowlees PM. The effectiveness of telemental health: a 2013 review. Telemedicine e-Health. 2013;19(6):444–54.
28. HLAA. COVID-19: guidelines for health care providers – video-based telehealth accessibility for deaf and hard of hearing patients. Hearing Loss Association of America; 2020.
29. C2C. Telehealth for providers: what you need to know. 2021.
30. ATA. Practice guidelines for video-based online mental health services; 2013.
31. Hom MA, Weiss RB, Millman ZB, Christensen K, Lewis EJ, Cho S, et al. Development of a virtual partial hospital program for an acute psychiatric population: Lessons learned and future directions for telepsychotherapy. J Psychother Integr. 2020;30(2).

The Teleclinician

5

Hossam Mahmoud, Omar Elhaj,
and Marlene McDermott

The term teleclinician refers to any healthcare professional delivering BHS remotely, including psychiatrists, psychiatric nurse practitioners, psychiatric physician assistants, psychologists, clinical social workers, marriage and family therapists, and clinical professional counselors, to name a few. Practicing as a teleclinician does not require formal training or particular certification in telehealth. Rather, the "tele" designation is meant to indicate the medium of delivering care and that the clinician is delivering BHS remotely through ICT.

As we have seen in previous chapters, a TBH program is ideally built on a successful match between the teleclinician, OS, and patient population. The teleclinician's ability to deliver high-quality care will require not only clinical competency, but also tech-savviness and cultural competency that would enable them to develop rapport with patients, despite geographic distance [1]. In this chapter, we provide some practical guidance for

H. Mahmoud (✉)
Tufts University School of Medicine, Boston, MA, USA

O. Elhaj
Case Western Reserve University School of Medicine,
Cleveland, OH, USA

M. McDermott
Array Behavioral Care, Mount Laurel, NJ, USA
e-mail: marlene.mcdermott@arraybc.com

H. Mahmoud et al. (eds.), *Essentials of Telebehavioral Health*,
https://doi.org/10.1007/978-3-030-97325-4_5

69

teleclinicians to consider before, during, and after the session. Since program considerations for facility-based services were covered in Chap. 3, this chapter will focus on home-based services in outpatient settings.

Prior to Sessions

In the case of home-based TBH practices, OS support staff are typically not available. In this case, scheduling and other administrative tasks can be managed by the teleclinician providing services or their virtual support staff. Accordingly, teleclinicians may consider hiring their own administrative or clinical staff to support their TBH practice. They may also consider incorporating automated systems to assist with operations such as intake processes, paperwork, scheduling, and billing, to name a few.

Build an Online Profile

For home-based services that mirror in-person private practice, teleclinicians should consider creating an online professional profile that describes their training, scope of practice, treatment philosophies, and professional areas of interest. Such online profiles would assist patients as they navigate TBH service options to find teleclinicians that align with their treatment needs [2].

Appropriateness for TBH

As mentioned in Chap. 4, there are no absolute patient contraindications for assessing or treating patients through TBH. Rather, deciding who can be well served through TBH services, and under which circumstances, is largely a clinical decision [3], whereby the teleclinician determines and recommends appropriateness for individual patients [3]. Therefore, having clear screening guidelines for patients helps reduce treatment mismatch or incompatibility resulting from clinical acuity, connectivity issues, or inability to engage in BHS via ICT. Screening can be completed by the teleclinician or properly trained support or clinical staff, or through self-administered screening questionnaires that potential patients complete prior to treatment initiation.

Screening criteria vary depending on the type of TBH program or teleclinician's practice. Teleclinicians may consider patient acuity and whether their practice is able to meet the patient's needs. In considering clinical acuity, teleclinicians may look at symptom severity, functional impairment, and chronicity or persistence of symptoms, as well as previous response and adherence to treatment [4]. Screening criteria generally follow similar criteria to those that may prompt referral to in-person care, such as imminent risk of harm to self or others, severe psychosis and disorganization, or inability to engage with ICT. Examples of clinical scenarios that may prompt patient referral to in-person BHS are provided in Chap. 4. To emphasize, however, the decision on whether a patient should be referred out or not should be made by the teleclinician, in the context of the patient's needs and the resources available to the teleclinician and the OS to adequately support these needs.

Scheduling

Scheduling can be maintained by live staff via phone, synchronous messaging, or asynchronous messaging, or it can be driven by automated patient-navigated systems. A combination of these approaches is sometimes used. However, regardless of which scheduling system is used, appointment reminders such as the ones listed next are important and should be automated whenever possible:

- Text reminders to a patient's phone are important.
- Email messages have value but can often get missed in someone's email inbox or sent to spam.
- Reminders should be sent when the session is scheduled, and at least two other times before the session, one preferably within 24 h prior to the appointment.

Informed Consent and Patient Information

It is standard practice to obtain signed informed consent before starting treatment. Different jurisdictions have variations in the required content to be included and communicated through the informed consent process. Such variations may include whether verbal consent is acceptable and whether electronic signatures for written consent are allowed [3], to name a few. Therefore, be cognizant of jurisdiction-specific regulations and use informed consent agreements that are specific to the jurisdiction where the patient is located [1]. A checklist of suggested components commonly included in informed consent forms is given in Toolbox 5.1. A more comprehensive example of the components of an informed consent and patient information form is also provided in Chap. 4.

In addition, a HIPAA Notice of Privacy Practices (see Chap. 3 for reference) must be provided to all patients prior to their first session. The U.S. Department of Health & Human Services (HHS) has issued Model Notices of Privacy Practices, with examples that can be accessed through the following website on "Model Notices of Privacy Practices": https://www.hhs.gov/hipaa/for-professionals/privacy/guidance/model-notices-privacy-practices/index.html.

It would also be helpful to include guidance on appropriate patient setup as part of the informed consent and patient information process, and on your website or patient portal that is readily accessible to patients.

Because of the value of collaboration with other treating clinicians when delivering services through TBH, make sure to collect the contact information of the patient's primary care provider (PCP) and other healthcare clinicians involved in their care. Also, consider obtaining release of information (ROI) forms signed by the patient to allow communication with these clinicians as standard practice. Finally, collect the contact information of the patient's emergency contact or other support contact(s) and obtain a signed ROI form in case communication with them is needed.

The American Academy of Child and Adolescent Psychiatry (AACAP) provides resources and templates on consent for treatment, patient information, ROI, and other practice management templates that can be found at https://www.aacap.org/aacap/Clinical_Practice_Center/Business_of_Practice/Practice_Forms_HIPAA_Disclosures.aspx.

Toolbox 5.1 Informed Consent Checklist
- Comply with jurisdiction-specific laws
- Mirror the components of an in-person informed consent
- Provide patient educational resources on ICT
- Provide guidance on appropriate patient setup

Also include the following in the informed consent form:

- Type and scope of services
- Program or practice structure
- Privacy, confidentiality, and ICT security
- Scheduling
- Documentation
- Billing
- Potential risks, including tech failure
- Emergency planning
- Mandatory reporting
- Teleclinician availability between sessions
- Appropriate circumstances for contact between sessions
- Teleclinician response time
- No-show policy

Technological Preparedness

TBH services rely on seamless communication through reliable ICT with little to no disruptions. For this reason, it is pivotal that you ensure technological preparedness from your patient's side and from your side to minimize technological disruptions and to have backup plans to address such disruptions if they arise [1, 2]:

- Ensure that your videoconferencing software, computer operating system, and web browser are up to date, particularly for browser-based videoconferencing platforms.
- Consider that despite their security value, some firewalls may interfere with some types of web traffic.
- Pre-test your Internet speed before rolling out services, and before starting your sessions on a given day, especially if you suspect or anticipate possible Internet disruptions. Internet speed tests can be done via https://www.speedtest.net/.
- If using a call-enabled device, such as a smartphone for TBH, place it on Do Not Disturb mode as the videoconferencing can be interrupted by phone calls.
- Always have a backup plan for tech failures and always communicate that plan to your patients during the first session. This includes having backup Internet connection, such as through mobile hotspots, and backup laptops, tablets, or phones.
- Make sure you have easy access to patients' phone numbers in case of a technology disruption.
- If you do have technological support through a help desk, make sure you always have their contact information readily available.
- It is highly recommended to offer a practice session to patients prior to their first clinical appointment in order to help familiarize them with the ICT and troubleshoot any related problems [5]. That can also address possible patient concerns about using ICT in healthcare delivery and privacy issues.

Crisis Planning

Crisis management for clinically supervised settings is discussed in Chap. 3. For home-based services in clinically unsupervised settings, develop protocols for both medical and BH emergencies. What constitutes a BH emergency in TBH typically mirrors in-person care, with the added potential for technology-related disruptions. Examples may include but are not limited to suicidal ideations, self-harm thoughts, homicidal ideations, aggression thoughts, inability to care for self, worsening depressive symptoms, manic symptoms, or psychotic symptoms. They may also include allergic reactions, medication side effects, and medication toxicity.

Crisis management protocols vary depending on the jurisdiction, teleclinician's comfort, patient population, and in-person resources. Nevertheless, we recommend you consider incorporating the following into your crisis management protocol:

- Be familiar with the mental health code, including civil commitment laws in the jurisdictions where your patients are located [3].
- Request that the patient enters the physical address of their location at the time of the session, as a change in location may change emergency management protocols [2].
- Ensure you have ready access to the patient's phone number and that of their emergency contact.
- Ensure you are familiar with healthcare facilities, including EDs, in the patient's geographic area, and have ready access to their contact information.
- Even though many jurisdictions may not require an ROI in emergencies, it is good practice to have signed ROI forms on file for communication with identified PCPs and other healthcare professionals involved in your patients' care, or with identified family members, significant others, or social support systems, including the "patient support person" (PSP).
- A PSP can be a friend, family, or community member identified by the patient to assist in emergencies, such as suicide risk. The teleclinician may then contact the PSP for assistance in assessing the emergency or possibly initiating emergency service calls from the patient's location [3].
- Communicate the emergency protocol to patients in writing prior to sessions [5].

Teleclinician Setup

Consider both your office and the patient's room a "patient exam ination room." Thus, keep a professional background the same way you would if you were seeing patients in your office and maximize ambiance and comfort in your setup [5]. As such, we recommend that you:

- Dress and groom professionally, and avoid clothing or wall picture with patterns and colors that may be distracting on video.
- Ensure that your setup is private and that conversations with patients or clinical discussions with other healthcare professionals cannot be overheard [5]. Make sure the same privacy standards apply to your patients also.
- Your camera and your patient's camera should ideally be at the eye level, and in a manner that enables both faces to be clearly visible [5].
- Minimize light from windows or lighting from behind you or your patient; rather, top lighting is preferred [2].
- Reduce any background noise and consider using microphones and noise-canceling headsets, both for privacy and audio clarity.
- Avoid identifiers that include your exact address or other personal information.
- Minimize distractions to you by turning off or muting phones (unless being used in session) and turning off notifications and reminders on your device.
- Minimize distractions to the patient by avoiding repetitive behaviors that might cause noise or interfere with the audio quality, such as tapping pens or shuffling papers.
- If an unexpected intrusion occurs, consider going on mute while you address the issue, after informing the patient of the interruption.
- Pre-test your setup prior to starting your sessions for the day [5].

During Sessions

The Basics

For facility-based services, patients typically check in to see their teleclinician at the OS the same way they check in for in-person care. The OS staff will typically obtain pertinent patient information, such as identity verification, contact information, emergency contact, preferred pharmacy, and payment information. The OS staff can also provide patients with information about the name, biography, and credentials of the teleclinician.

For home-based services, the teleclinician must collect the above-described patient information, verify the patient's location at the start of every session, and learn the location of the in-person facility closest to the patient location. Depending on how you decide to set up your practice, patients may be asked to submit a scanned copy of a government-issued photo identification form when signing up for services or asked to show such proof of identification on camera during their first session [2]. In addition, the teleclinician should make available their full name, credentials, qualifications, license number, and other registration numbers when applicable [2].

During the first session:

- Start by introducing yourself and verifying the patient's identity.
- Describe your office setup and general location.
- Verify the patient's location and the privacy of their environment.
- Make sure to discuss with the patient TBH as a method of BHS delivery that may be new to them; for patients with previous experience with TBH, inquire about how their past experience was [5, 6].
- Make sure to address any patient concerns about PHI security, privacy, and confidentiality [6]. Share with your patient your privacy and security measures, and encourage them to always be in a private secure location for sessions.

- Review the informed consent form with the patient and make sure to discuss safety and crisis management, as well as the potential for terminating services if it is deemed that the patient cannot be safely or effectively treated virtually [3].
- Make sure to discuss your therapeutic framework and to set treatment expectations and boundaries [6]. There should be mutual commitment to that framework, including connecting from a private quiet space, not connecting from a moving vehicle, not recording sessions without written permission, dressing appropriately for sessions, and handling interruptions [5]. In addition, discuss expectations and boundaries regarding substance use, particularly immediately prior to or during sessions.
- Outline the emergency protocol, which should have been provided to the patient in advance in writing to ensure patient understanding.
- Review boundaries and expectations regarding communication in between sessions, including the management of emergencies that may occur in between sessions [6]. In addition, work with the patient to identify a PSP who can be contacted to assist with emergencies.

Rapport and Therapeutic Alliance

Teleclinicians should consider the impact of the use of ICT and the remote nature of TBH service delivery on rapport with their patients [3]. The literature shows that therapeutic alliance can be successfully maintained with TBH. Teleclinicians must make an active effort to create a welcoming ambiance and engaging session. A frank discussion about the patient's concerns regarding virtual care and a willingness to work through any ICT-related frustration can help maintain a strong alliance [5]. While the first session with your patient can entail several discussions on the therapeutic framework, make sure to express interest, convey professionalism, and demonstrate empathy. This is best achieved with the following recommendations:

- Be consistent in your sessions, including timeliness, setup, and ambiance.

- Describe your office space and ask the patient to describe their space. For example, ask where patients live, who they share their space with, and their neighborhood.
- Conduct yourself in a professional manner [5], starting with your background and office setup, grooming, attire, and language.
- Be patient and courteous as your patients familiarize themselves with operating ICT and develop comfort with remote care delivery. Well-placed humor and humility, especially in the face of technical challenges, could go a long way to ease your patient's potential anxiety or discomfort.
- Maintain eye contact while shifting your gaze between the screen and the camera in order to be able to see the patient [5]. The farther you are from your monitor and camera, the less noticeable gaze shifting is. The ideal distance is about 2 feet. Remember to look at the camera to demonstrate attention and eye contact. Avoid looking solely at the screen as this gives the impression that you are looking away from the patient and may give the impression that you are disinterested or unengaged. If your video platform allows, place the patient's video image directly under your camera for best eye contact.
- For home-based services, use the window that TBH offers into the patient's personal space as an opportunity to build rapport.
- Avoid interruptions during sessions.
- Do not check your phone, email, or texts during sessions, as that can be distracting and can convey lack of engagement.

Clinical Considerations

While clinical practice with TBH is similar to in-person care, some areas require special attention due to the remote nature of the work and the use of ICT. Some signs and symptoms of BH conditions may be difficult to detect using videoconferencing, and therefore might go unnoticed [7]. This may include mild substance use effects, subtle changes in cognition or orientation, involuntary movements, including tics and tremors, and poor hygiene [5]. Recognizing these challenges, teleclinicians should:

- Practice in a manner that is collaborative. When delivering services into an OS, make sure to incorporate input from the OS staff, including case managers, psychotherapists, physicians, and patient navigators. For home-based services, collaborate with patients' PCPs, psychotherapists, and other healthcare professionals involved in their care [2, 3, 8].
- Be particularly attentive to verbal and nonverbal cues [5].
- Particularly with home-based services, take advantage of the fact that TBH can provide a window into the patient's personal space, including indications of organization, environmental factors, and even engagement in hobbies.
- Ask the patient questions about symptoms or signs that you are unable to assess remotely. For example, if poor hygiene was reported or identified as a current issue or as a warning sign that predicts worsening of symptoms, routinely ask about the patient's hygiene practices.

Technological Issues

Even with technological preparedness, your connectivity, hardware, or software may experience issues. If the videoconferencing session unexpectedly fails, attempt to troubleshoot by following these steps:

- Call your patient and inform them that you are attempting to identify and fix the technological issue.
- Test your Internet connection.
- Ensure all browser cookies are clear.
- Log out and back in.
- And, yes, attempt to restart your device!
- Contact you help desk, when available.
- If efforts to reconnect via videoconferencing fail, follow the protocol discussed and agreed upon with your patient. This usually includes switching to phone sessions until the issue is resolved [5], but different facilities and teleclinicians may have other policies and procedures. In addition, some payers may

have reimbursement restrictions on the use of audio-only communication for delivering treatment.

- Consider rescheduling the session if clinically appropriate.

Crisis Management

For facility-based services, involve the OS staff as per crisis management protocols developed and communicated within the OS. This is covered in more detail in Chap. 3. For home-based services, attempt to manage early indication of crisis in a manner similar to in-person sessions, including attempts at risk assessment, de-escalation, safety planning, and resource identification. With TBH, it is recommended you adopt the following approaches for safety and crisis management:

- Ensure the physical location of the patient during the session is verified at the beginning of each session.
- Avoid sessions while the patient is in a vehicle, even when parked, as that will limit your ability to assist them during a crisis. If unavoidable, ask for the vehicle's location, make, model, and license plate number.
- Involve emergency contacts, such as the PSP or another identified emergency contact to assist with crisis management.
- If an ED assessment is needed and the PSP able to accompany the patient, call the emergency department in advance.
- If the PSP or other support is not available, consider calling local emergency services.
- If emergency services are needed, use www.usacops.com, a county-based link to police departments in the United States, or www.policelocator.com, which allows searching by city name.
- Throughout the crisis, keep the session open while contacting resources and keep the patient informed of whom you are contacting and involved in managing the situation.
- Depending on your assessment of the crisis and your patient's clinical needs, as well as your therapeutic alliance, determine the degree and details of information to share with the patient

with regard to crisis management and emergency service involvement.

- Consider recommending or facilitating involuntary hospitalization, knowing the variations that exist by jurisdiction.

Prescribing

Prescribing best practices in TBH align with in-person care. As such, it is advisable to:

- Prescribe while in session to ensure pharmacy information is accurate and verify that the prescriptions have been sent to the pharmacy.
- Prescribe in accordance with federal and local jurisdiction laws, including those that regulate the prescribing of controlled substances.
- Enroll in the jurisdiction-specific prescription monitoring program and to check the database prior to prescribing certain controlled substances, as it is considered best practice and in some jurisdictions a legal requirement to do so.
- Familiarize yourself with e-prescribing software options, including those for prescribing controlled substances, and utilize only one e-prescribing program for consistency and continuity of care. Preference is for a program with EHR integration capabilities. A database of e-prescribing software can be found at https://surescripts.com/network-alliance/eprescribing-prescriber-software.

Ending the Session

- Summarize the treatment plan and make sure the patient has a clear understanding of it and that their questions or concerns are addressed.
- Consider any potential safety issues and a corresponding safety plan, be it pertaining to the patient's safety or to that of the OS staff as the session is ending [3].

- If prescribing medications, confirm to the patient that their medication has been prescribed, including name, dose, quantity, and refill. Make sure that the patient knows where to get their prescription filled.
- Set up a follow-up appointment, which can be scheduled by the teleclinician or the OS support staff, depending on the setting and already-established workflows.
- Especially after the first few sessions, it is recommended at the end of the session to seek the patient's feedback about their experience and identify any areas for improvement.

After Sessions

Documentation

Documentation should be completed as close to the time of the session as possible. OS facilities likely have their own time frame requirements for completing documentation, as well as requirements and templates on how BHS, including TBH sessions, are documented. Documentation should be conducted in accordance with federal and jurisdiction-specific laws, and such records must be stored in a manner that complies with HIPAA and HITECH [2].

Some teleclinicians prefer to start documenting during the session, which can improve efficiency but may also have its drawbacks. If your preference is to do concurrent documentation during the session, it is important to ensure that documenting does not distract you from conducting the session in a meaningful and engaged manner. Make sure that documenting does not require looking away from the camera for a significant period of time as that may give the impression that you are disinterested or unengaged. Furthermore, looking away from the video portion of the screen may run the risk of missing your patient's nonverbal cues. Finally, repetitive keystroke sounds can be distracting or bothersome to patients, so if you are documenting during the session, make efforts to shield patients from such sounds, possibly using a microphone that is placed further away from the keyboard.

Having documentation templates may improve efficiency. While clinical documentation templates vary by facility, healthcare setting, and teleclinician, the APA has provided guidance on the components of clinical documentation for TBH sessions. This can be accessed at https://www.psychiatry.org/psychiatrists/practice/telepsychiatry/toolkit/clinical-documentation.

As mentioned in Chap. 3, for TBH service delivery, EHR is preferable over paper charting. In addition to clinical documentation, EHR charts should include patient identification and demographic information, contact information, copy of informed consent, patient information forms, and insurance and billing information [2]. A database of EHR software can be found at https://surescripts.com/network-alliance/eprescribing-prescriber-software.

Documentation is further discussed in Chap. 3.

Clinical Collaboration

While cross-specialty collaboration is considered good clinical practice in general, it becomes particularly important for home-based services. To ensure the delivery of high-quality care, collaborate with your patients' PCPs, psychotherapists, and other healthcare professionals involved in their care [2, 3, 8]. In addition to the fact that care coordination can support better patient care, such collaborative relationships may prove critical during emergencies [2]. Separately, these relationships also serve as an antidote to remedy the professional isolation some teleclinicians experience.

Facility-based TBH services tend to be collaborative. For example, vital signs are usually obtained and reported by the OS staff. For home-based services, when vital signs are necessary, teleclinicians may consider the following options:

- Relying on measurements from equipment that patients have at home (blood pressure cuffs, thermometer, scale).
- Supplying basic equipment to patients (e.g., a blood pressure cuff).

- Using local pharmacies, with vital sign testing options.
- Relying on clinical data obtained from a patient's other health-care providers [8].

Coding and Billing

Reimbursement for TBH by public and private payers requires proper coding and billing procedures. Familiarize yourself with the most up-to-date version of the Current Procedural Terminology (CPT) codes applicable to your scope of practice and the services you provide. Historically, teleclinicians have used the same CPT codes used for in-person care, with a code modifier that indicates that the service was delivered remotely. Recognizing that the reimbursement landscape is constantly evolving, consult with professional societies, CMS, and private

Toolbox 5.2 Billing and Reimbursement Resources
- The Centers for Medicare and Medicaid Services https://www.cms.gov/Medicare/Medicare-General-Information/Telehealth
- American Psychiatric Association https://www.psychiatry.org/psychiatrists/practice/tele-psychiatry/blog/apa-resources-on-telepsychiatry-and-covid-19
- American Psychological Association https://www.apa.org/monitor/2020/06/covid-telepsychology
- Center for Connected Health Policy https://www.cchpca.org/

payers regarding reimbursement requirements and CPT codes for TBH in order to stay up to date with the latest regulations (see Toolbox 5.2). For more information on additional resources for clinical, professional, regulatory, and reimbursement guidelines, see Toolbox 5.3.

> **Toolbox 5.3 Resources on Clinical, Professional, Regulatory, and Reimbursement Guidelines for TBH**
>
> - *American Psychiatric Association.*
>   - Telepsychiatry toolkit.
>   https://www.psychiatry.org/psychiatrists/practice/telepsychiatry/toolkit
>   - Telemental health guide.
>   https://www.psychiatry.org/psychiatrists/practice/telepsychiatry/blog/apa-and-ata-release-new-telemental-health-guide
> - *American telemedicine association.*
>   - ATA practice guidelines for video-based online mental health services.
>   https://pubmed.ncbi.nlm.nih.gov/32897476/
> - *Centers for Medicare and Medicaid Services.*
>   - Medicare telemedicine health care provider fact sheet.
>   https://www.cms.gov/newsroom/fact-sheets/medicare-telemedicine-health-care-provider-fact-sheet
>   - Quality measures: Traditional MIPS requirements.
>   https://qpp.cms.gov/mips/quality-requirements

Beyond Sessions

Ethical Considerations

Teleclinicians must maintain the same degree of ethical and professional guidelines when practicing TBH as for in-person care. This pertains to issues of consent, patient rights, patient autonomy, strict privacy practices, and clear professional boundaries [3]. This also requires following jurisdiction-specific guidelines on ethical training required for licensure and ethical practices such as duty to report and to notify.

Teleclinician Well-Being

TBH has the potential to remedy certain factors that contribute to teleclinician burnout. For example, TBH may improve the teleclinician's sense of control over their schedule since it alleviates the burden and time of commuting to a healthcare facility or office, or in between different practice locations. This time can instead be spent on social or family activities, self-care or sleep, all factors that mitigate burnout. Alternatively, this time can be used to address practice management needs such as quality assurance initiatives, administrative tasks, and documentation [9].

On the other hand, TBH practice may pose certain challenges. This includes the risk of professional and academic isolations, social isolation, and a possible sense of alienation from the OS. In addition, some teleclinicians, specifically telepsychiatrists, have voiced concerns about the potential of TBH to blur the boundaries between workplace and home life, to create pressure to work longer hours or be available after hours [9]. TBH may also be associated with a more sedentary lifestyle, which may itself have burnout and health implications [9].

One other issue that became widely discussed among clinicians after the rapid transition to TBH in the context of the COVID-19 pandemic has been the feeling of sensory overload during TBH videoconferencing sessions due to numerous reminders, pings, and popups, be it due to emails, instant messages, or texts. These repeated notifications can cause distractions during sessions, making it difficult at times to fully engage with patients and causing some teleclinicians to feel distracted and overwhelmed. This issue also has the potential to impact patient care due to "alert fatigue," which refers to situations where clinicians may fail to appropriately respond to safety alerts due to becoming desensitized to the sheer volume of such alerts [10]. Accordingly, while minimizing distractions conveys respect and engagement to the patient, it may also mitigate burnout and the potential negative outcomes of alert fatigue.

Our recommendations for teleclinicians are as follows:

- Remember to take care of yourself!
- Establish clear boundaries with your employer or OS, regarding schedule, work hours, and after-hours availability. Communicate these boundaries clearly with OS staff.

- Consider delegating some practice management tasks to support staff as administrative tasks can be stressful and time consuming [11].
- During sessions, minimize distractions by turning off or muting phones (unless being used for patient communication) and turning off notifications and reminders on your device.
- Make sure to allow a few minutes in between sessions, which you could use to stand up and stretch your muscles, or to look away from the monitor so that you avoid chronic eye strain.
- Develop personal goals to ensure family life and social life are protected and involve family and friends in discussions about these goals. You may have to make a more concerted effort to plan social activities and engage in personal interests.
- Consider models of TBH that require collaboration and close interactions with other clinicians and OS staff to mitigate academic, social, and occupational isolation.
- Consider diversifying your work by combining clinical practice with research or academia [9] and by participating in professional organizations and societies.
- Remember to exercise regularly or maintain an active lifestyle.
- Invest in or request ergonomic office furniture for optimal spine support.
- Finally, remember that there are many resources to support clinicians on the issues of well-being and burnout [9] (see Toolbox 5.4).

Toolbox 5.4 Resources on Well-Being and Burnout
- American Psychiatric Association
  https://www.psychiatry.org/psychiatrists/practice/well-being-and-burnout
- The National Academy of Medicine
  https://nam.edu/systems-approaches-to-improve-patient-care-by-supporting-clinician-well-being/
- American Medical Association
  https://www.ama-assn.org/practice-management/physician-health/6-big-things-must-change-beat-physician-burnout

References

1. Mahmoud H, Whaibeh E, Mitchel B. Ensuring successful telepsychiatry program implementation: critical components and considerations. Curr Treatment Opt Psychiatry. 2020.
2. ATA. Practice guidelines for video-based online mental health services;2013.
3. Shore JH, Yellowlees P, Caudill R, Johnston B, Turvey C, Mishkind M, et al. Best practices in videoconferencing-based telemental health April 2018. Telemedicine e-Health. 2018;24(11):827–32.
4. Zimmerman M, Morgan TA, Stanton K. The severity of psychiatric disorders. World Psychiatry. 2018;17(3).
5. Lopez A, Schwenk S, Schneck CD, Griffin RJ, Mishkind MC. Technology-based mental health treatment and the impact on the therapeutic alliance. Curr Psychiatry Rep. 2019;21.
6. Mahmoud H, Whaibeh E, Mitchell B. Ensuring successful telepsychiatry program implementation: critical components and considerations. Curr Treatment Opt Psychiatry. 2020;7(2):186–97.
7. Mahmoud H, Vogt EL, Sers M, Fattal O, Ballout S. Overcoming barriers to larger-scale adoption of telepsychiatry. Psychiatric Ann. 2019;49:82–8.
8. Daniel H, Sulmasy LS. Policy recommendations to guide the use of telemedicine in primary care settings: an American College of Physicians Position Paper. Ann Intern Med. 2015;163(10).
9. Vogt EL, Mahmoud H, Elhaj O. Telepsychiatry: implications for psychiatrist burnout and well-being. Psychiatr Serv. 2019;70(5):422–4.
10. AHRQ. Alert Fatigue. Agency for healthcare research and quality. 2019.
11. Mahmoud H, Naal H, Mitchel B. Evaluating a multicomponent strategy to address burnout, job engagement, and job satisfaction among telepsychiatrists. J Psychiatr Pract. 2021

Information and Communication Technologies

Bridget Mitchell and Hossam Mahmoud

Information and Communition Technologies (ICT) includes both the software and hardware used to deliver care remotely, including videoconferencing platforms and other communication methods used between teleclinicians and patients and between teleclinicians and other healthcare professionals. ICT can also include web-based applications, smartphone applications, EHR systems, and e-prescribing programs.

With so many options for ICT, it is the type of TBH services to be delivered and the other OPTIC components that should guide the choice of ICT. It should factor in the OS resources, patient population's needs and familiarity with technology, the teleclinician's scope of practice, and the cultural and regulatory factors shaping technology use in remote healthcare delivery. It is important to balance the ICT requirements of your TBH program with cost, utility, and ease of use (see Toolbox 6.1). The rapid advancement of technological innovations has been paired with a gradual decrease in the cost of more basic ICT software and hardware, such as computers, phones, applications, e-prescribing programs,

B. Mitchell
Compass Health Center, Northbrook, IL, USA

H. Mahmoud (✉)
Tufts University School of Medicine, Boston, MA, USA

© The Author(s), under exclusive license to Springer Nature
Switzerland AG 2022
H. Mahmoud et al. (eds.), *Essentials of Telebehavioral Health*,
https://doi.org/10.1007/978-3-030-97325-4_6

Toolbox 6.1 ICT Checklist

- Ensure compliance with federal HIPAA and HITECH requirements
- Familiarize yourself with state or other jurisdiction privacy laws
- Have clear processes for documenting, retrieving, and storing PHI in accordance with regulatory requirements
- For facility-based services, follow OS procedures and policies to ensure electronic data security and hardware security
- For home-based services, develop procedures and policies to ensure electronic data security and hardware security
- Patient communication media include HIPAA-compliant videoconferencing, patient portals, telephone, and text-based software
- Clinician communication media include videoconferencing, EHR, encrypted email, and electronic fax
- Choose EHR and e-prescribing for documentation and prescriptions
- Connectivity: at least 5 Mbp in upload and download speeds

and videoconferencing platforms. While innovations and advances in ICT features and specifications may be appealing, advanced ICT may end up being unnecessary for your particular TBH practice, excessively costly and more difficult to use. This can result in poor engagement and utilization and compromise the cost-effectiveness and sustainability of the TBH program.

Regardless of equipment or program, all ICT programs and platforms used to deliver TBH services in the United States must comply with HIPAA and HITECH requirements for the protection, storage, and sharing of PHI. In addition, state or other jurisdiction PHI privacy and data security laws should be followed, keeping in mind that they may vary from federal laws [1]. These regulations apply to both facility-based or home-based TBH services, whether synchronous or asynchronous, and regardless of clinical setting [2, 3]. The APA and ATA recommend that organizations have procedures and policies to ensure electronic data security and hardware security and that both organizations and teleclinicians have clear processes for documenting, retrieving, and storing TBH records [1]. Keep in mind that the rapid adoption of TBH that took place during 2020 in the context of the COVID-19 pandemic led to a significant increase in the "digital footprint" of BHS and concomitantly to an increase in the "attack surface." This has created data vulnerability for teleclinicians, facilities, and patients, such as data theft vulnerabilities and malware security issues [4] and highlights the importance of continued vigilance when it comes to cybersecurity in TBH. It also emphasizes the need to conduct regular training on ICT use, HIPAA, HITECH, and cybersecurity for the teleclinician and all staff involved in supporting the TBH program.

ICT choices should ensure a balance between the quality, efficiency, user experience, and accessibility of the service on one hand, and the cost of hardware, software, Internet connectivity, staff training, and technology support on the other [6]. For facility-based TBH practice, consider the already existing infrastructure and its ability to incorporate and maintain newly added ICT. Two approaches have been followed: (1) the facility develops and implements its own TBH ecosystem by getting its own hardware, software, Internet connectivity, and needed tech support, building on the business model it has established for in-person care, or (2) the facility uses a third-party vendor to assist with ICT solutions [6]. This second option is at times needed with smaller healthcare facilities that may not have the experience or technological support for implementing TBH programs. Example 6.1 discusses

Example 6.1 ICT Preparedness
An example of ICT preparedness of a TBH program that
delivers direct patient care for medication management is
presented in the publication "Planning and Implementing
Telepsychiatry in a Community Mental Health Setting: A
Case Study Report," [5] which can be accessed through
https://pubmed.ncbi.nlm.nih.gov/32897476/. In this case
study, a TBH program in a community mental health setting
describes the use of ICT, including

- HIPAA-compliant videoconferencing platform for delivering TBH sessions.
- EHR system for documentation
- e-Prescribing for sending prescriptions
- Electronic fax for receiving testing results
- HIPAA-compliant encrypted email for communication between OS staff and teleclinician

ICT preparedness was further enhanced through teleclinician and staff training on backup procedures in the case of technological breakdown. It also included the use of

- An Internet hotspot in case of Internet connectivity issues
- Backup laptops fully charged in case of loss of electric power or failure of primary hardware

ICT preparedness and provides an example of a healthcare organization partnering with a vendor for clinical and technological support.

Software

Patient-facing software for delivering TBH sessions includes videoconferencing platforms, patient portals, and smartphone applications and text-based software. Non-patient-facing software includes programs and platforms for internal communication, documentation, and other clinical operations. While there is likely some overlap with the software used for delivering TBH sessions, non-patient-facing software may also include the use of EHR systems, encrypted email, and electronic fax to communicate and coordinate care among treatment team members, including the OS support staff, other clinicians, pharmacies, laboratories, and other testing centers [1, 6].

Over the past few years, several HIPAA-compliant platforms have become available to deliver TBH videoconferencing sessions. The cost to use these platforms has significantly decreased, and some are available for use by teleclinicians at no cost to them. So when considering your options, ensure that the videoconferencing platforms and applications selected have the necessary security and verification parameters appropriate for TBH services [1]. Privacy specifications require that the videoconferencing connection be via point-to-point encryption. Federal Information Processing Standards (FIPS) are the recognized standards for cybersecurity and encryption for what would be considered acceptable levels of security [7]. Current encryption standards must meet "FIPS 140-2 certified 256 bit standard." When reviewing options for HIPAA-compliant platforms, note that many vendors may require a Business Associate Agreement (BAA) for ensuring HIPAA compliance. The APA recommends contacting the vendor to verify what such an agreement entails and any potential effects on your practice [8].

Oftentimes, software programs will prompt users to accept and initiate updates in order to ensure the programs are working optimally or enable upgrades to existing features. If working with an OS, the information technology (IT) team of the site should offer guidance on when to accept these updates and should also make users aware of upcoming updates that must be completed in order for programs to function optimally. At times, maintenance may need to be performed on these programs, and IT teams should work with teleclinicians and OS staff to ensure that this maintenance is scheduled for a time where system access is not needed. In the event that the software programs experience a disruption, IT should document these instances, both in order to inform affected parties of the disruption and temporary workflow changes that may be necessary and to be able to assess for patterns or triggers that may predict these outages. For teleclinicians seeing patients at home and without access to an IT team, similar considerations should be factored into decisions around when to implement necessary software updates.

The California Association of Marriage and Family Therapists offers resources on TBH software, including HIPAA-compliant platforms at https://www.camft.org/Resources/Legal-Articles/Telehealth-HIPAA-and-Compliant-Telehealth-Platforms.

Hardware

Hardware choices are informed by the resources of the facility, physical setting, and needs of the patient population. At the basic level, TBH can be delivered using a camera-enabled and microphone-equipped secure laptop, tablet, or smartphone connected through a robust secure Internet connection to another camera-enabled microphone-equipped secure laptop, tablet, or phone. Beyond that, many hardware variations exist. For example, in an OS with larger patient rooms, larger monitors might be needed to improve patient experience, whereas in smaller rooms, a computer monitor or laptop screen would be sufficient. In addition, while virtual reality equipment might offer a positive user experience for patients, they are not considered necessary to deliver TBH, and their costs continue to be prohibitive [9].

The choice of hardware is also informed by the types of software chosen for delivering TBH services. Such software choices, including for videoconferencing platforms, EHR systems, and e-prescribing programs, may dictate the choice of optimal operating system and compatible hardware, on the teleclinician's end and the OS or patient's end. For example, some platforms require computers, while others require smartphones or tablets for an optimal user experience. Some platforms require particular operating systems, which may rely on specific brands of hardware equipment. Others may offer more versatility and allow the teleclinician and patient to choose between a variety of devices.

Hardware components should be assessed on a regular basis for functionality, including routinely testing the speakers, microphones, and cameras prior to sessions and replacing nonfunctional equipment as needed. It is also important to have backup equipment in case of sudden breakdown. We recommend that the teleclinician and OS routinely test their hardware briefly at least once a week, to ensure sessions can be completed without delay or interruption. Teleclinicians seeing patients in their homes should advise patients to test their equipment prior to a scheduled session to ensure they can see, hear, and be heard when meeting with the teleclinician. Most videoconferencing platforms allow users to pre-test the platform's functionality and necessary hardware, to ensure participants are able to communicate seamlessly during sessions.

All hardware and software access must be protected with robust passwords that should be changed at regular intervals; computers and other devices must be set to auto-lock after a period of inactivity, usually no more than 15 minutes, with re-authentication requirements for unlocking. This decreases the risk of a security breach due to unauthorized access. Multifactor authentication is highly encouraged and, whenever available, should be used. Consider using biometric security programs, such as facial recognition or fingerprint, for an added layer of security [10].

Hardware must be stored in a secure manner to prevent unauthorized access. While the portability of devices such as laptops, tablets, and smartphones has increased convenience, teleclinicians must securely store these devices when not in use. Secure physical storage is still necessary, even with robust password protections for such devices. This applies to both home-based and facility-based TBH services. For equipment at the OS, the staff must ensure that similar storage safeguards are in place for all equipment used to deliver TBH sessions or to store or transmit PHI. Devices used to deliver TBH services must not be shared with unauthorized users [7]. In addition, these devices should have a functionality to allow them to be remotely disabled, locked, or wiped in case of theft or loss [7]. Should repairs be needed at any point for the hardware of either the teleclinician or the OS, care should be taken in securing all PHI to avoid unauthorized access during the course of repair.

Toolbox 6.2 ICT Security Recommendations
- Use robust passwords and change them regularly
- Consider using auto-lock after inactivity
- Consider using multifactor authentication for added security
- Consider using biometric security software (e.g., facial recognition, fingerprint recognition)
- Ensure hardware is safely stored and well-secured
- Do not use shared devices or allow others to use the devices you use for TBH
- Make sure personal firewall and antivirus software are updated (up-to-date security patches)
- Conduct regular training on HIPAA, HITECH, and cybersecurity for the teleclinician and all staff involved in the TBH program

The security and access of TBH delivery devices should be regularly monitored (see Toolbox 6.2) [11]. These devices should have updated personal firewall and antivirus software, as well as the most up-to-date security patches [7, 11, 12]. In addition, avoid installing software applications that are not necessary for delivering services [11] as they may slow down your machine and may increase security risks.

Any incidents where security has been compromised, such as unauthorized access to PHI, should be reported, reviewed, and documented as per the individual facility's compliance processes and security protocols. An incident autopsy must be initiated, and depending on the type and magnitude of the breach, an incident may have to be reported to state agencies or HHS [3, 11]. Any identified vulnerabilities pertaining to the security breach would have to be addressed through enhancement of security processes to avoid future breaches [11].

A cybersecurity checklist can be found at https://www.healthit. gov/sites/default/files/basic-security-for-the-small-healthcare-practice-checklists.pdf.

CMS Rules on Security, Privacy, and Breach Notification can be found at https://www.cms.gov/outreach-and-education/medicare-learning-network-mln/mlnproducts/downloads/hipaaprivacyandsecuritytextonly.pdf.

Connectivity

Secure and reliable broadband Internet connection is essential for the delivery of seamless TBH services [6]. TBH requires sufficient bandwidth to support the quality of the audio and video during sessions. Typically, this requires upload and download speeds of at least 5 Mbp to avoid frequent buffering, delays, and pixelation [8]. Speed tests can be tested at www.speedtest.net.

If using a computer, we highly recommend a hardwired Internet connection, e.g. Ethernet, with a direct connection between the computer and the Internet service provider's modem to minimize connectivity disruptions [7]. Secure wireless Internet can be used, especially with mobile devices, such as tablets and smartphones, but the risk of signal fluctuation may affect the strength of the connection, thereby compromising the quality of the audio and video transmission.

Remember that the quality of the videoconferencing session relies on the connectivity and bandwidth on both the teleclinician's end and the patient's end [7]. This is coordinated with the OS staff for facility-based services. For home-based services, inform patients of best practices for connectivity, as well as preferred software or hardware for a good videoconferencing experience [7].

Contingency Planning

Technology breakdown may occur due to software, hardware, or connectivity problems, which may cause session disruptions. Therefore, a backup plan should be developed and clearly communicated in advance to OS staff, teleclinician, and patient. While this plan may involve switching to a telephone session [1], it should also cover rescheduling and prescribing policies in case the sessions cannot be completed. Technology preparedness is covered in Chap. 5.

References

1. Shore JH, Yellowlees P, Caudill R, Johnston B, Turvey C, Mishkind M, et al. Best practices in videoconferencing-based telemental health April 2018. Telemedicine e-Health. 2018;24(11):827–32.
2. CDC. Health insurance portability and accountability act of 1996 (HIPAA). Center for Disease Control and Prevention. 2018.
3. HHS. HITECH Act Enforcement Interim Final Rule. U.S Department of Health & Human Services. 2017.
4. HPHS. Health industry cybersecurity - securing telehealth and telemedicine. Healthcare and public health sector coordinating counsils. 2021.
5. Mahmoud H, Whaibeh E, Mitchell B. Ensuring successful Telepsychiatry program implementation: critical components and considerations. Curr Treatment Opt Psychiat. 2020;7(2):186–97.
6. Mahmoud, H., Naal, H., Cerda, N. Planning and implementing telepsychiatry in a community mental health setting. Community mental health journal. 2020;1–7.
7. ATA. Practice guidelines for video-based online mental health services; 2013.
8. APA. Platform and software requirements. American Psychiatric Association.
9. Aboujaoude E. Telemental health: why the revolution has not arrived. World Psychiatry. 2018;17(3).
10. Mahmoud H, Vogt EL, Sers M, Fattal O, Ballout S. Overcoming barriers to larger-scale adoption of telepsychiatry. Psychiatric Ann. 2019;49:82–8.
11. Healthit. CYBERSECURITY The protection of data and systems in networks that connect to the internet. Health IT. 2010.
12. NCMW. The psychiatric shortage causes and solutions. National Counsil for Mental Wellbeing. 2018.

Cultural and Regulatory Context

7

Hossam Mahmoud, Emile Whaibeh,
and Marlene McDermott

Cultural Considerations

One of the main advantages of TBH is its ability to eliminate the physical distance between patients and providers. In fact, many TBH practices have been specifically designed to target underserved communities and populations with poor access to BHS [1, 2]. This wide geographic distance prompts considerations pertaining to possible cultural differences that may arise and underscores the necessity of delivering culturally appropriate care. For instance, a teleclinician from an urban area and working with remote populations has to take many factors into consideration: Patients might come from communities with stronger kinship bonds, more economic woes [3, 4], and specific BH problems related to history of marginalization, deprivation or oppression [5]. Moreover, patients from remote or rural communities may experience more mental health stigma and lower help-seeking

H. Mahmoud (✉)
Tufts University School of Medicine, Boston, MA, USA

E. Whaibeh
Department of Public Health, Faculty of Health Sciences,
University of Balamand (UOB), Beirut, Lebanon

M. McDermott
Array Behavioral Care, Mount Laurel, NJ, USA
e-mail: marlene.mcdermott@arraybc.com

101

H. Mahmoud et al. (eds.), *Essentials of Telebehavioral Health*,
https://doi.org/10.1007/978-3-030-97325-4_7

behavior, potentially due to privacy concerns in their "small, tightly knit" community settings [5, 6].

However, marginalization is certainly not exclusive to rural communities; underserved populations exist in various settings and include people whose access to care is impeded by systemic barriers of an economic, cultural, or linguistic nature [7] or pertaining to other demographic characteristics, including ethnicity, age, social status, educational level, sexual and gender identity, and history of chronic conditions or disabilities [8, 9]. As the demographic makeup of the United States continues to change and the ethnic, linguistic, and cultural diversity continues to grow [10], cultural considerations will only become more relevant over time. It follows that the likelihood of a teleclinician working with a patient who may not speak the same language or share the same history or culture will only increase moving forward. Moreover, an increase in the clinician's cultural competence has been linked to an increase in patient satisfaction, information seeking, information sharing, and treatment adherence [11, 12]. Cultural factors influence the development of trust and mitigation of mistrust and concerns about stigma [1]. Accordingly, it is strongly recommended that teleclinicians receive training on geographic, social, and cultural competency, especially for the populations they are likely to serve [13].

Culture and Behavioral Health

Culture is defined by the DSM-5 as the "systems of knowledge, concepts, rules, and practices that are learned and transmitted across generations" [14]. This includes one's language, religion, spirituality, family structures, life-cycle stages, ceremonial rituals, and customs, as well as moral and legal systems. Understanding the interplay between culture on behavioral health is crucial for the following reasons. First, culture shapes perceptions and expressions of mental illness, so much so that what is deemed pathological in one culture may be understood to be standard in another. For instance, when it comes to migrants who have escaped oppressive regimes, it is not uncommon to have thoughts that may appear as paranoid to a clinician from a different background [14]. Different cultural groups even vary in the way they define BH-related constructs, such as "normality," "distress," and "abnormality." Second, culture also shapes populations' attitudes toward people with BH conditions and beliefs about treatment and health-seeking behavior [15]. For instance, some traditional Chinese American and First Nation cultures depend on traditional medicine, herbs, or rituals for healing in lieu of or in addition to standard BHS. Third, for TBH specifically, culture plays a role in the relationship of certain communities and populations with technology use; this can explain the differences in acceptance, access, and diffusion of technology across different cultures [16]. For example, a study conducted by Jefee-Bahloul et al. [17] with Syrian refugees in Turkey found that only 45.7% of the participants reported acceptance of TBH with the most cited reasons for a negative response being concerns about Internet security and preference to receive the services face-to-face. The study also found that women were significantly more likely to accept face-to-face psychiatry than men. It was also found that they were less likely to accept TBH compared to their male counterparts, albeit without statistical significance. According to the authors, this could be due to gender-based cultural differences; women within this culture tend to be more conservative and less likely to engage in public interactions altogether. This could also explain their hesitancy toward using BHS, in general, and TBH service, in particular, by virtue of perceiving them as less secure [18]. Similarly, in the United States, there are documented differences between various ethnic groups regarding their interest in, access to, attitudes toward, and experiences with ICT, which undoubtedly affect TBH service delivery [19]. Therefore, cultural considerations for beliefs and attitudes on BH and BHS, including stigma, should be incorporated into the planning and implementation of TBH services to support the delivery of culturally appropriate care.

Culturally Appropriate Care

Culturally appropriate virtual care was defined by Yellowlees et al. in 2008 [19] as the delivery of BHS that are "guided by the cultural concerns of all racial or ethnic groups, including psychosocial background, typical styles of symptom presentation, immigration histories and other cultural traditions, beliefs and values." A limitation of such a definition is that it may appear to restrict culture to ethnicity and race, as Elizabeth Brooks et al. explain in Myers and Turvey's book, *TBH: Clinical, Technical, and Administrative Foundations for Evidence-Based Practice*. Therefore, the authors proposed to broaden the definition to include "any group of individuals with distinct customs, beliefs, values, histories, and communication styles." Cultural competence refers to the process by which individuals and systems integrate and transform their knowledge about groups and communities into specific standards, best practices, policies, and attitudes to increase the quality of services and produce better health outcomes [20]. Training on cultural competence should include (1) appreciation for the role of culture in shaping perceptions, attitudes, and behaviors vis-à-vis BH conditions and BHS, (2) acceptance and respect of cultural variations and valuing diversity, (3) effective incorporation of culturally adapted practices, and (4) continuous focus on self-awareness of personal biases and cultural influences [21].

A four-step plan that can be followed by institutions interested in being more intentional about culturally appropriate TBH care is provided in Fig. 7.1. It is worth noting that there is no one-size-

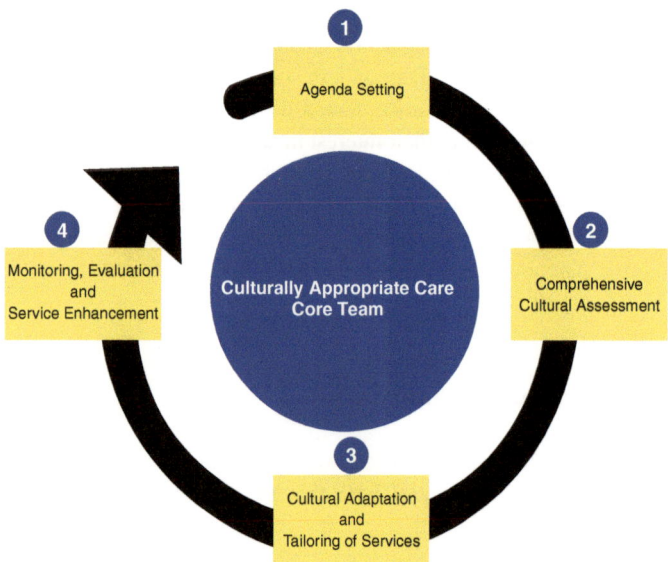

Fig. 7.1 Four-step plan for culturally appropriate TBH care

fits-all solution when it comes to a component as complex, multidimensional, multifaceted, and ever-changing as culture.

1. Agenda Setting

The first step toward enhancing the cultural appropriateness of your program or practice is to recognize the influence of culture on BH and BHS delivery and allocate a sufficient amount of resources for the leadership and program personnel to develop their cultural competence. Even though top-down approaches are often scrutinized, having the support and commitment of the organization or program leadership can be instrumental in facilitating the process. First, identify key stakeholders and assemble a group that would constitute the core team of your agenda setting. The composition of the core team largely depends on the available personnel, the type and size of the institution, and the amount of available resources. Broadly, the core team needs to include (1) physicians, nurses, and administration and support personnel from the OS, (2) consultant teleclinician(s), (3) ICT professional(s) familiar with the available technological infrastructure of the community and OS, and (4) key informants and representatives from the patient population, community, or culture of interest. Be mindful of the makeup of the core team and the power dynamics within it. Make sure everyone's input is represented, and no voices are sidelined or ignored as this would defeat the purpose of this exercise.

The core team is then tasked to set the agenda for the organization by (1) developing strategies or multiphase multiyear work plans for the organization to enhance the cultural appropriateness of care, (2) providing guidance on cultural and administrative concerns, and (3) writing the mission statement and the goals of the organization, highlighting the aim of increasing reach, improving acceptance, and gaining the trust of the community of interest. Area leaders, such as community organizers, sovereign tribal entity leaders, tribal councils, and respected elders, can be a great asset to your core team. Due to their dual role as vital members of the community and as strategic planners in the TBH service offering site, they can be uniquely poised to voice the concerns of their community and make recommendations for your practice that inform service design and future evaluation efforts. Moreover, they are able to become BH champions within their own communities, increasing the knowledge and acceptance of their fellow community members of BHS, and TBH in particular. They ensure that the community's concerns surrounding TBH services are well-understood by teleclinicians and the OS personnel.

2. Comprehensive Cultural Assessment

Now that your organization has taken the initiative to become more culturally competent, a comprehensive cultural assessment is necessary. The core team is tasked to determine the cultural indicators of interest (see Toolbox 7.1) and design or select the appropriate tools to assess them in order to have a deeper understanding of the local community they aim to serve. If you are in the planning stage, this is a crucial step because it offers insight on which aspects of a TBH program may work and which may not go over well with the target patient population. To this end, you could conduct focus group discussions and interviews can be conducted with local BH clinicians, former or current patients who received BHS at the OS, local mental health activists, community leaders, and key informants. A comprehensive cultural assessment also entails looking critically at your own OS staff and teleclinicians to become aware of the cultural diversity that exists within your own practice or program and to inquire about the cultural development needs that your personnel and how you could support them. The purpose of such activities is not simply to gather data about your population of interest; rather, it is about utilizing this cultural knowledge to develop a long-term strategy with measurable outcomes to incorporate culture into your program's principles, policies, and practices. In plainer terms, the best way to understand what a community needs and wants is by simply asking them.

Toolbox 7.1 Suggested Checklist of Factors for Culturally-Appropriate Care
- Patient population's geographic location and area infrastructure
- History of major events in the region, including natural disasters
- Linguistic, religious, and ethnic characteristics

- For refugee and immigrant populations, countries, languages and cultures of origin
- History of collective trauma and systemic racism, such as First Nations and African Americans
- Other relevant social determinants of health
- Variations in social norms and expectations about treatment, such as with rural communities
- Variations in stigma across communities and subgroups within communities
- Variations in access, attitudes, and usage of ICT
- Existence of linguistically validated screening tools
- Cultural fit between teleclinician and patient population
- Necessity for further cultural competency training or refresher sessions
- Necessity for administrative and institutional policy changes to improve access

Following this exercise, the core team needs to convene to synthesize the newly acquired cultural knowledge, extract preliminary findings, set priorities, identify areas of enhancements, and make recommendations that would guide the development of the TBH program. As culture is a cross-cutting issue, we recommend organizing the recommendations around the five core components of the OPTIC acronym: (1) recommendations pertaining to the OS structure, policies, workflows, and staff, (2) recommendations regarding cultural, linguistic, and socioeconomic barriers faced by the patient population, (3) clinical recommendations for the teleclinicians (see Toolbox 7.2), (4) recommendations pertaining to cultural attitudes vis-à-vis ICT use, and (5) recommendations regarding changing cultural norms and attitudes through knowledge and awareness-raising and advocacy efforts. For further assurance, the findings could be shared once again with representatives from the community via individual consultations or town-hall-style community meetings to validate the findings and acquire more feedback from the community on the generated recommendations. The final document is then circulated with the advisory board of the institution for comment and approval before proceeding to the implementation phase.

Toolbox 7.2 Further Resources on Culturally-Appropriate Care

Professional societies and associations have developed guidance for delivering culturally competent care:

- American Psychiatric Association. Best Practice Highlights for Treating Diverse Patient Populations https://www.psychiatry.org/psychiatrists/cultural-competency/education/best-practice-highlights
- American Psychiatric Association. Cultural Formulation Interview (2013) http://www.multiculturalmentalhealth.ca/wp-content/uploads/2013/10/2013_DSM5_CFI_InformantVersion.pdf
- American Psychiatric Association. Cultural Formulation Interview Supplementary Modules 2013 http://www.multiculturalmentalhealth.ca/wp-content/uploads/2013/10/2013_CFI_supplementarymodules.pdf
- National Association of Social Workers. Standards and Indicators of Cultural Competence in Social Work Practice 2015 https://www.socialworkers.org/LinkClick.aspx?fileticket=PonPTDEBrn4%3D&portalid=0
- American Psychological Association. Guidelines for Providers of Psychological Services to Ethnic, Linguistic, and Culturally Diverse Populations 2017 http://www.apa.org/pi/oema/resources/policy/provider-guidelines.aspx
- American Counseling Association. Code of Ethics 2014 https://www.counseling.org/resources/aca-code-of-ethics.pdf
- U.S. Department of Health and Human Services (2018). National Standards for Culturally and Linguistically Appropriate Services (CLAS) in health and healthcare Retrieved from https://www.thinkculturalhealth.hhs.gov/clas

3. Cultural Adaptation and Tailoring of Services

The third step of the plan is to translate the generated knowledge into concrete solutions and put it into practice (see Example 7.1). The core team, preferably with the assistance and guidance of a TBH consultant, should lead the cultural adaptation process of TBH services. Cultural adaption begins at the recruitment level with the inclusion of diverse groups of people from the community in every level of the organization's structure, especially in leadership and decision-making positions. Cultural competency requirements should be explicit in the job descriptions to help foster a welcoming and safe work environment, especially for racial, ethnic, linguistic, and cultural minority applicants. Major pitfalls to avoid are tokenism, paternalism, and unequal and unfair representation in decision-making roles. Second, cultural adaptation requires diversity training for the existing and newly hired OS staff and teleclinicians. Even if the OS personnel are local to the region or community, some training might still be necessary. It is worth noting that even though diversity training is important, it cannot be an isolated one-time occurrence; this would not yield any meaningful cultural change at the organization level. Diversity training should be done regularly and meaningfully and supported by institutional and administrative policy changes, that reinforce respectful conduct and deter harmful actions. Moreover, cultural adaptation entails tailoring your services and developing new services to address needs previously unrecognized or misunderstood. Respectful and effective communication with the population of interest, partnerships with local organizations with strong ties with the community, and hiring new staff members such as interpreters or TBH outreach workers are all examples of steps that your program can undertake to ensure the provision of culturally appropriate services.

Example 7.1 TBH for a First Nation Tribal Community

First Nation Tribal communities often face unique challenges in accessing care. In addition to instances where the population is remotely located, intergenerational trauma and cultural views that embrace a more holistic attitude toward medicine and healing may result in skepticism toward care provided to the community by outsiders. In addition to these cultural nuances, tribal laws and practices may influence the ways in which medical or BHS are accessed. The authors of this chapter had to consider these aspects when establishing TBH programs with tribal populations who wanted to offer BHS within their community clinics. In an effort to support culturally appropriate care, a member of the tribal community was recruited to help train both teleclinicians and program support staff on aspects of culturally appropriate care for tribal populations, including an acknowledgment of the unique histories of each tribe and prevailing attitudes toward BHS, healthcare services in general, and medications. Where possible, this was supplemented with on-site visits by the teleclinician to the OS, to both orient the teleclinician to the tribal community and culture, meet with community leaders and staff, and help establish trust between the teleclinician and the community whom they would be serving.

Teleclinicians should have cultural competency that allows them to approach their patient populations in a manner that is culturally appropriate [9]. Approaches to deliver culturally appropriate care may include self-educating on the culture, geography, and environment of the patient population, conducting on-site visits to OS whenever possible, and using cultural facilitators when needed [22]. Teleclinicians should explore a patient's experience and comfort with technology overall and with receiving care via ICT [22]. Understanding these factors within the context of TBH can play an instrumental role in enhancing patient engagement and ultimately treatment success. Cultural facilitators can be used for training on the environment and culture of the patient population [23]. Such cultural training opportunities have been documented to help facilitate culturally appropriate TBH services, especially for First Nation communities [24].

4. Monitoring, Evaluation, and Service Enhancement

The value ascribed to a TBH intervention largely depends on the program or practice's ability to assess the effectiveness of services to patients, communities, funding agencies, and decision-makers [25]. Moreover, the evaluation of TBH programs has moved beyond patient satisfaction with the remote services and has shifted to issues such as feasibility, reliability, cost-effectiveness, and improved clinical outcomes [25]. Culturally speaking, the purpose of Monitoring and Evaluation (M & E) is to collect relevant data on patient, teleclinician, and OS staff attitudes and behaviors in response to the cultural adaptation measures undertaken. Data on patient satisfaction, access, engagement, technology, and other variables are used to monitor, evaluate, and improve the program and it cultural adaptation [1]. For more details on specific measures and indicators related to the monitoring and evaluation of TBH programs, refer to Chap. 8. Finally, this step facilitates future strategic planning as it tests the impact of the cultural adaptations incorporated into the TBH program and subsequently informs the future directions and further adaptations for the program [25].

Regulatory Considerations

The regulatory framework that shapes the delivery of TBH includes the guidelines, regulations, and laws that guide the delivery of BHS with those that regulate the remote delivery of health-care services. This means that prior to delivering TBH services teleclinicians must familiarize themselves with the clinical practice regulations of the jurisdiction where the OS or patients are located [26]. For example, different jurisdictions have different mental health codes that dictate the practice of BH care, especially in BH emergencies that may require involuntary holds, duty to warn, and reporting requirements [26]. In addition, federal and jurisdiction-specific regulations govern the practice of remote care delivery, placing requirements for licensure, conditions for establishing a patient–clinician relationship, and restrictions on prescribing controlled substances. When federal and jurisdiction regulations differ, the more stringent regulation should be followed. For example, HIPAA and HITECH are federal laws that regulate the protection, storage, and communication of PHI. If a state or other jurisdiction has more stringent regulations governing BH patient privacy or the transmission of BH health information, the more stringent regulations are to be followed [27].

The Ryan Haight Act

The Drug Enforcement Agency (DEA) oversees the prescribing of controlled substances, whether in person or online [28]. To be able to prescribe controlled substances legally, every prescribing clinician is required to register with the DEA. This registration alone was not enough to stop the inappropriate prescribing of controlled substances through online prescribing [28]. Therefore, a federal law, the Ryan Haight Online Pharmacy Consumer Protection Act, was passed in 2008 to ensure the patients who are receiving the controlled substances are appropriately diagnosed with the conditions that warrant a controlled substance prescription. The Ryan Haight Act aimed to address the irresponsible distribution of controlled substances via online pharmacies. A consequence of the Ryan Haight Act was that it made it illegal to prescribe controlled substances without the prescriber first having an in-person evaluation with the patient unless the conditions for one of seven exceptions are met (see Toolbox 7.3) (Levine & Wein 2020). While the act addressed issues related to the unregulated distribution [29] and diversion of controlled substances, it failed to take into consideration TBH services delivering appropriate care. As a result, an in-person patient evaluation became a necessary condition for authorized teleclinicians to be able to prescribe controlled substances. Subsequent in-person follow-up visits at intervals of no more than 3 months also became necessary to continue prescribing controlled substances [30].

Outside of the Veterans Affairs system [3], the two exceptions most commonly utilized in TBH for the prescribing of controlled substances remotely were (1) having a licensed health professional involved in treating the patient be present while the prescribing teleclinician is evaluating the patient and (2) having the patient located at an OS that is a DEA-registered facility.

Another exception to the Ryan Haight Act [5] allows prescribers to prescribe controlled substances via telehealth in case of a national emergency [29]. This is what happened when the COVID-19 pandemic was declared a public health emergency in March 2020, temporarily permitting the prescribing of controlled substances across a variety of settings and OS, including for home-based TBH services, until the state of emergency is lifted [31].

Toolbox 7.3 The Seven Exceptions to In-Person Visit Requirement for the Ryan Haight Act of 2008 for Telehealth Practices [32]

1. If the patient is in an office with a healthcare professional who is treating the patient and that patient receives care via telehealth (e.g., patient receiving a TBH session with a psychiatrist while at a primary care office)
2. If the patient is located inside a DEA registered hospital or clinic and completes a telehealth visit
3. If clinician is an employee or contractor of Veteran's affairs
4. If the service is of Indian Health Service or tribal organization
5. If there is a public health emergency, as declared by the Secretary of Health and Human Services
6. If the prescriber has been approved for a special registration
7. If there is a Department of Veterans Affairs medical emergency

Finally, the Special Registration for Telemedicine Act was signed into law in 2018 to allow telehealth prescribers a special registration to lawfully prescribe controlled substances without a first in-person examination [32, 33]. The Special Registration would constitute exception (6) of the Ryan Haight Act [32]. While the DEA was given directives to create the guidelines for the special registration, with an October 2019 deadline [32], these guidelines have not been published at the time of writing this book.

Licensure

The jurisdiction in which the patient is located is considered the jurisdiction of BHS delivery [22]. Accordingly, when the patient and teleclinician are located in different jurisdictions, the teleclinician is required to be licensed in the jurisdiction where the patient is located [26]. Exceptions include certain federal systems, such as the Department of Defense and Department of Veterans Affairs, as well as Indian Health Service, all of which may allow practicing with one license across multiple states or jurisdictions [26].

While many TBH services tend to be delivered in one jurisdiction, some TBH programs, particularly within larger healthcare systems, may serve multiple OS in different jurisdictions. This usually requires teleclinicians to obtain multiple licenses [26] depending on the OS locations, which can be a cumbersome process. Some solutions have been put in place to ease the burden of obtaining multiple professional licenses. For instance, some states offer special telehealth licensure to practice beyond state lines. In addition, some US states and territories have joined the Interstate Medical Licensure Compact to offer an expedited pathway to physician licensing [22, 26].

Delivering TBH under multiple professional licenses means having to comply with the clinical practice regulations governing BHS and TBH service delivery in multiple jurisdictions, depending on where the OS are located [26]. Having multiple professional licenses also requires keeping up with continuing education requirements, which may vary significantly across different states.

Reimbursement

Historically, reimbursement limitations were considered a barrier to implementing TBH programs. Prior to the COVID-19 pandemic, Medicare had geographic restrictions that limited reimbursement for telehealth services to designated facility-based OS in rural and BH clinician shortage areas. While most Medicaid plans included telehealth benefits, there were many variations when it came to reimbursement by private payers [26]. In response to the public health emergency, the Centers for Medicare & Medicaid Services (CMS) suspended the OS restrictions, allowing reimbursement for home-based TBH services [31]. In addition, executive orders and legislations in several jurisdictions that passed during the pandemic expanded or required reimbursement for telehealth services, sometimes at parity with in-person care [34]. The TBH reimbursement landscape is constantly evolving, so it is important to ensure the following:

- Verify TBH reimbursement regulations and requirements on a regular basis and stay up to date on the latest information pertaining to telehealth reimbursement eligibility.
- Maintain proper documentation and coding practices, with the appropriate billing codes and modifiers to indicate services were delivered via TBH.
- Inform your patients of billing practices, TBH reimbursement eligibility, and any pertinent financial charges to the patients [8].
- Discuss a payment method and cadence with patients during intake.

Collaborative Agreements

Nurse practitioners looking to deliver TBH services should familiarize themselves with how the jurisdiction's regulations and laws impact their practice. A clear understanding of practice environments is necessary due to the variations that exist among states, districts, and territories when it comes to nurse practitioner practice, ranging from restricted to reduced, to full unrestricted practice [35].

Ensure that you have a clear understanding of any requirements for collaborative agreements, prescriptive delegations, and supervision in the jurisdiction where the patient is located. Such requirements may dictate a cadence for meetings with the collaborating physician, modes of communication, oversight requirements, and the type of activities that are needed to meet collaboration or supervision requirements. Some states also have limits on the number of nurse practitioners with whom a physician is permitted to enter a collaborative agreement [36].

State-by-state information on collaboration and supervision requirements for nurse practitioners can be found at https://www.aanp.org/advocacy/state/state-practice-environment.

References

1. Hilty DM, Gentry MT, McKean AJ, Cowan KE, Lim RF, Lu FG. Telehealth for rural diverse populations: telebehavioral and cultural competencies, clinical outcomes and administrative approaches. mHealth. 2020;6.
2. Moreno FA, Chong J, Dumbauld J, Humke M, Byreddy S. Use of standard webcam and internet equipment for telepsychiatry treatment of depression among underserved Hispanics. Psychiatr Serv. 2012;63(12).
3. Dwyer JW, Lee GR, Coward RT. The health status, health services utilization, and support networks of the rural elderly: a decade review. J Rural Health. 1990;6(4).
4. Phillips CD, McLeroy KR. Health in rural America: remembering the importance of place. Am J Public Health. 2004;94(10).
5. Nicholson LA. Rural mental health. Adv Psychiatr Treat. 2008;14(4).
6. Aisbett D, Boyd C, Francis K, Newnham K, Newnham K. Understanding barriers to mental health service utilization for adolescents in rural Australia. Rural Remote Health. 2007;7(1).
7. Brooks E, Turvey C, Augusterfer E. Provider barriers to telemental health: obstacles overcome, obstacles remaining. Telemed e-Health. 2013;19(6).
8. ATA. Practice guidelines for video-based online mental health services; 2013.
9. Mahmoud H, Whaibeh E, Mitchell B. Ensuring successful Telepsychiatry program implementation: critical components and considerations. Curr Treatment Opt Psychiat. 2020;7(2):186–97.

10. Colby S, Ortman J. Projections of the size and composition of the US population: 2014 to 2060. Curr Popul Rep. 2015.

11. Paez KA, Allen JK, Beach MC, Carson KA, Cooper LA. Physician cultural competence and patient ratings of the patient-physician relationship. J Gen Intern Med. 2009;24(4).

12. Roncoroni J, Tucker CM, Wall W, Nghiem K, Wheatley RS, Wu W. Patient perceived cultural sensitivity of clinic environment and its association with patient satisfaction with care and treatment adherence. Am J Lifestyle Med. 2014;8(6).

13. Mahmoud H, Sers M, Tuite J. Enhancing telemental health for rural and remote communities. Becker's Health IT. 2018.

14. APA. Cultural formulation. In: Diagnostic and statistical manual of mental disorders. 5th ed. Washington, DC: American Psychiatric Association; 2013.

15. Cheon BK, Chiao JY. Cultural variation in implicit mental illness stigma. J Cross-Cult Psychol. 2012;43(7).

16. Brooks E, Manson SM, Bair B, Dailey N, Shore JH. The diffusion of Telehealth in rural American Indian communities: a retrospective survey of key stakeholders. Telemed e-Health. 2012;18(1).

17. Jefee-Bahloul H, Moustafa MK, Shebl FM, Barkil-Oteo A. Pilot assessment and survey of Syrian refugees' psychological stress and openness to referral for telepsychiatry (PASSPORT study). Telemed e-Health. 2014;20(10):977–9.

18. Jefee-Bahloul H. Telemental health in the Middle East: overcoming the barriers. Front Public Health. 2014;2.

19. Yellowlees P, Marks S, Hilty D, Shore JH. Using e-health to enable culturally appropriate mental healthcare in rural areas. Telemed e-Health. 2008;14(5).

20. Simmons CS, Diaz L, Jackson V, Takahashi R. NASW cultural competence indicators: A new tool for the social work profession. Journal of Ethnic & Cultural Diversity in Social Work. 2008;17(1):4–20.

21. Purnell L. Transcultural health care: a culturally competent approach. 4th ed. F.A. Davis Company; 2012.

22. Shore JH, Yellowlees P, Caudill R, Johnston B, Turvey C, Mishkind M, et al. Best practices in videoconferencing-based telemental health April 2018. Telemed e-Health. 2018;24(11):827–32.

23. Mishkind MC. Establishing telemental Heath Services from conceptualization to powering up. Psychiatr Clin N Am. 2019;42(4).

24. Kruse CS, Bouffard S, Dougherty M, Parro JS. Telemedicine use in rural native American communities in the era of the ACA: a systematic literature review. J Med Syst.

25. Hilty DM, Feliberti J, Evangelatos G, Lu FG, Lim RF. Competent cultural telebehavioral healthcare to rural diverse populations: administration, evaluation, and financing. J Technol Behav Sci. 2019;4(3).

26. Mahmoud H, Vogt EL, Sers M, Fattal O, Ballout S. Overcoming barriers to larger-scale adoption of telepsychiatry. Psychiatric Ann. 2019;49:82–8.

27. HHS. How do I know if a state law is "more stringent" than the HIPAA Privacy Rule? U.S Department of Health and Human Services. 2003.

28. Liang BA, MacKey T. Searching for safety: addressing search engine, website, and provider accountability for illicit online drug sales. Am J Law Med 2009;35(1).

29. Levine S, Wein E. COVID-19: DEA and SAMHSA guidance for treating opioid use disorders via telehealth. San Francisco: Newstex; 2020.

30. Huskamp HA, Busch AB, Souza J, Uscher-Pines L, Rose S, Wilcock A, et al. How is telemedicine being used in opioid and other substance use disorder treatment? Health Aff. 2018;37(12).

31. Whaibeh E, Mahmoud H, Naal H. Telemental health in the context of a pandemic: the COVID-19 experience. Curr Treatment Opt Psychiat. 2020;7(2):198–202.

32. Lacktman N. Prescribing controlled substances without an in-person exam: the practice of telemedicine under the Ryan Haight act. Becker's Health IT; 2017.

33. Acosta J, Lacktman N. President signs new law allowing telemedicine prescribing of controlled substances: DEA special registration to go live. Health Care Law Today. 2018.

34. Morse S. Telehealth to become permanent under trump executive order. Healthcare Finance. 2020.

35. AANP. State practice environment. American Association of Nurse Practitioners; 2021.

36. Board of Registered Nursing. Frequently asked questions regarding nurse practitioner practice. Sacramento; 2004.

Monitoring, Evaluation, and Quality Assurance

8

Bridget Mitchell, Hossam Mahmoud, and Hady Naal

Incorporating a Monitoring and Evaluation (M & E) framework into your Telebehavioral Health (TBH) program or practice supports not only quality assurance and improvement, but also long-term success and sustainability. M & E can facilitate tracking the progress toward meeting your program goals using identified measures, and can guide program modifications for improved outcomes. M & E can also be used to refine your program goals and the outcome measures used to track the progress toward such goals.

A sound M & E approach starts with reviewing historical data to establish baseline data points to contextualize the TBH program goals and guide the development of your program. M & E should span all the OPTIC components (see Chap. 1), including the Originating Site (OS), the patient population, the teleclinician, Information and Communication Technologies (ICT), and the

B. Mitchell
Compass Health Center, Northbrook, IL, USA

H. Mahmoud
Tufts University School of Medicine, Boston, MA, USA

H. Naal (✉)
Global Health Institute at the American University of Beirut, Beirut, Lebanon

Department of Public Health, University of Balamand, Beirut, Lebanon

© The Author(s), under exclusive license to Springer Nature Switzerland AG 2022
H. Mahmoud et al. (eds.), *Essentials of Telebehavioral Health*, https://doi.org/10.1007/978-3-030-97325-4_8

cultural and regulatory context. In general, data should be collected and tracked on a regular basis to identify patterns, challenges, strengths, and areas of growth within your TBH program. Approaches to data collection can be qualitative, quantitative, or mixed, and the method of collection, storage, analysis, and reporting will vary accordingly.

A review of different evaluation approaches for TBH programs published in late 2020 reported that evaluation methods varied significantly by program, with no gold standard outcome measure or approach being identified. For example, operational outcomes, (i.e. nonclinical outcomes), can include volume of patients served, number of sessions conducted, patient engagement, and wait-times, among others. Clinical outcomes may include changes in scores on specific assessments, in screening measures of symptoms, in laboratory results, or in hospital admissions or readmissions, to name a few [1]. While both nonclinical and clinical outcomes were reported in a nonstandardized manner, most evaluation approaches were short-term and included small sample sizes. In addition, little emphasis was placed on important feasibility outcomes like cost-effectiveness. Clinically, few evaluation approaches incorporated standardized clinical tools [1]. However, there are some available guidelines and many case studies on telehealth programs published in the literature, as well as some reviews on methods to evaluate TBH programs. In this chapter, we synthesize findings from those publications and organize them by OPTIC component, recognizing that some outcome measures may serve as indicators or proxy indicators for more than one OPTIC component. In addition, we provide M & E and quality assurance recommendations based on the experiences of the authors and editors in the field of TBH.

Originating Site

Although few standardized instruments exist, some commonly used M & E indicators for TBH programs are given in Examples 8.1 and 8.2.

Example 8.1 Evaluation of a TBH Program for Direct Patient Care

An example of M & E of a TBH program that delivers direct patient care for medication management is presented in the publication "Planning and Implementing Telepsychiatry in a Community Mental Health Setting: A Case Study Report," which can be accessed through https://pubmed.ncbi.nlm.nih.gov/32897476/. In this case study, a TBH program in a community mental health setting reports on operational and clinical outcome measures. These include the number of sessions completed, volume of patients served, patient-care hours, efficiency of services, show rates, and wait-times. Some of these data points are compared among teleclinicians and between teleclinicians and the in-person clinician. The case study also reports on patient satisfaction with TBH sessions, patient-reported medication adherence, and on whether patients felt that their questions and concerns were addressed.

Example 8.2 Evaluation of a TBH Program for Direct Patient Care and Consultation Services

An example of M & E of a TBH program that delivers direct patient care and consultation services is summarized in the publication "Using Continuous Quality Improvement to Design and Implement a Telepsychiatry Program in Rural Illinois," which can be accessed through https://ps.psychiatryonline.org/doi/10.1176/appi.ps.201900231. This report describes outcome measures for a multimodal, multisite TBH program that delivers direct patient care, asynchronous consults, and synchronous consults:

- For direct patient care: patient satisfaction (including net promoter score or NPS), wait-times, number of patients served, and number of sessions completed.
- For consultation services: utilization, turnaround times, perceived utility, and primary care physician satisfaction.

Wait-Time

Wait-time refers to the amount of time patients wait to be able to have a session with a teleclinician, including first-time appointments for new patients and follow-up time for established patients. Average wait-time can be examined for a specific specialty, a specific teleclinician type, a particular teleclinician, or the TBH program itself. Decreases in wait-time while the volume of your patients is steady or increasing may indicate that your TBH program is effectively expanding access to care. Monitor this indicator at regular intervals. We recommend capturing the average wait-time for services each month and reviewing this data for trends at least every 3 months [2].

Volume of Patients Served

This indicator is somewhat related to wait-time in that, presumably, a TBH program that reduces wait-time for services would correspondingly serve a higher volume of patients. However, it is also important to examine wait-times and number of patients served in the context of other data points, such as patient engagement with the program and clinical complexity. For example, if the clinical needs of patients are complex enough to require more frequent follow-up appointments, both wait-times and volume of individual patients served may be impacted as the frequent follow-up needs affect the teleclinician's ability to accommodate new patients. In other cases, limited support services at the OS may decrease teleclinician productivity, which would also impact wait-times and volume of individual patients served [3].

Originating Site Staff Satisfaction

OS staff can offer valuable insights about your program. Feedback on the TBH program, including insights into workflow, processes, and staff satisfaction, can be collected through quantitative or qualitative methods, such as semi-structured interviews and self-completed surveys [4].

Cost-Efficiency

Cost-efficiency is essential for the sustainability of the TBH program. The OS should plan for and monitor the following cost-effectiveness variables [5]:

- Cost of hardware, software, and connectivity
- Cost of licensure for EHR and e-prescribing programs
- Staffing costs if adding a telehealth navigator
- Cost of developing and implementing new workflows
- Training costs for OS staff and teleclinician on ICT, workflows, and protocols
- Funding sources, including payer mix of the patient population
- Implementing appropriate billing practices

Patient Population

Nonclinical Outcomes

Patient satisfaction has been the indicator surveyed most in TBH program evaluations [4]. While increasingly common, receiving care via TBH may be faced with initial resistance or skepticism from patients regarding the utility, quality, or ease of engagement in comparison with in-person care. Monitoring patient satisfaction provides valuable insights, regarding aspects of service delivery related to the teleclinician, technology, and OS staff and setup (for facility-based services) [4].

Other commonly used outcome measures include show rates and program attrition, which may serve to some extent as proxy indicators of patient satisfaction and patient engagement. A no-show occurs when a patient does not show up for a scheduled appointment or cancels after a deadline specified in the cancellation policy of the OS or the teleclinician. A no-show should be distinguished from a proactive cancellation, whereby the patient cancels or reschedules an appointment in accordance with the cancellation policy. Attrition is when patients drop out of treatment with a program or a clinician. Average no-show and attrition rates for your TBH program can be compared to historical rates or concurrent rates for either in-person Behavioral Health Services (BHS) or for a comparable teleclinician at your OS. Such a comparison can provide valuable information on patient engagement and satisfaction and should prompt further examination of any contributing factors. For example, show rates and attrition rates may be more favorable due to the convenience of TBH services, the ability of a particular teleclinician to engage patients, or an enhanced sense of privacy that can assist in mitigating stigma [6]. On the other hand, show rates and attrition rates may be less favorably impacted by dissatisfaction with the technology, difficulty using ICT (especially for home-based services), or limited rapport with the teleclinician.

Given the multitude of factors that may affect show rates and attrition rates, it is important to survey your patients regularly through brief measures to prevent research fatigue. Patient feedback may be captured after each session through a short survey directly after completion of a session or at checkout in order to improve response rates. Ideally, the survey should be brief and should address satisfaction with the teleclinician, technology, OS setup, BHS, and session overall. While a short quantitative survey may increase response rates, there is value in obtaining more detailed insights from patients through qualitative surveys as well, although this may happen at longer time spans with smaller samples.

Clinical Outcomes

The clinical effectiveness of TBH has been demonstrated in the literature, with TBH clinical outcomes being comparable to in-person care [7, 8]. However, clinical outcomes have been less studied and less utilized in TBH program evaluation compared to nonclinical outcomes [1]. Both teleclinician assessment and Patient-Reported Outcome Measures (PROMs) have been used to monitor clinical outcomes for TBH programs. While there is significant value to monitoring symptom reduction through clinician assessments and clinical interviews, standardizing approaches may be more effective for more comparable and standardized tracking of clinical outcomes. These include using self-reported standardized clinical tools such as the Patient Health Questionnaire-9 (PHQ-9) for depressive symptoms, Generalized Anxiety Disorder Assessment (GAD-7) for anxiety symptoms, and Health-Related Quality of Life (HRQL) for global well-being, among other tools that have demonstrated psychometric evidence of validity and reliability.

Other clinical outcome measures may include laboratory testing for medication levels to monitor medication adherence and safety. This can also include tracking side effects of some medications, such as metabolic side effects, liver enzyme changes, and EKG changes. Finally, they can also monitor progress in SUD recovery, such as alcohol levels and urine drug screens.

At a population health level, clinical outcomes can include the impact of TBH programs on patient healthcare utilization and follow-up, for a clearly defined patient population, such as by a geographic area, catchment area, or insurance plan coverage. This includes tracking rates of Emergency Department (ED) utilization and admission rates to higher levels of care, such as Intensive Outpatient Programs (IOPs), Partial Hospitaization Programs (PHPs), residential programs, and inpatient hospitalizations. Other indicators can include possible impact on rates of outpatient follow-up after discharge from an ED or higher level of care [1].

Teleclinician

Indicators of success related to the teleclinician typically mirror those for in-person clinicians. These can include productivity, efficiency, quality of care provided, and patient satisfaction. Evidently, there is also significant overlap with the M & E indicators covered under the OS and patient population sections in this chapter. This section will highlight two aspects of M & E for teleclinicians: quality assurance and teleclinician satisfaction.

Quality Assurance

There are already established practice standards for BHS and TBH, outlined by professional societies and healthcare agencies (Example 8.3). However, different facilities and clinicians may choose to monitor quality using their own specific indicators and approaches for M & E. Clinical quality and quality of clinical documentation can also be assessed using peer reviews [4]. Peer reviews include evaluating the clinical work of a "peer" who has the same clinical specialty, and comparable credentials and scope of practice. Peer reviews assess the teleclinician's performance and quality of practice, against clearly identified criteria, usually through a review of the health record. Some commonly utilized quality criteria in peer reviews include

- Maintenance of accurate medication lists
- Documentation of care or treatment plan
- Documentation of diagnoses
- Use of DSM-5 criteria and diagnoses
- Documentation of risk and safety assessment

Example 8.3 Evaluation of Teleclinician Satisfaction and Engagement
An example M & E of teleclinician satisfaction and engagement is summarized in the publication "Evaluating a Multicomponent Strategy to Address Burnout, Job engagement, and Job Satisfaction Among Telepsychiatrists" [10]. In this report, a healthcare organization examined individual and organizational-level indicators such as teleclinician Net Promoter Score (NPS), retention rates, and output (hours worked per month), in addition to qualitative data. The report outlines a strategy to improve these teleclinician-associated indicators, contributing to improved NPS, retention rates, and hours worked per month over the period of time during which the strategy was implemented.

Resources on clinical, professional, regulatory and reimbursement guidelines for TBH

- **American Psychiatric Association:**
  - Telepsychiatry Toolkit
    https://www.psychiatry.org/psychiatrists/practice/telepsychiatry/toolkit
  - Telemental Health Guide
    https://www.psychiatry.org/psychiatrists/practice/telepsychiatry/blog/apa-and-ata-release-new-telemental-health-guide
- **American Telemedicine Association**
  - ATA practice guidelines for video-based online mental health services
    https://pubmed.ncbi.nlm.nih.gov/32897476/
- **Centers for Medicare and Medicaid Services**
  - Medicare Telemedicine Health Care Provider Fact Sheet
    https://www.cms.gov/newsroom/fact-sheets/medicare-telemedicine-health-care-provider-fact-sheet
  - Quality Measures: Traditional MIPS Requirements
    https://qpp.cms.gov/mips/quality-requirements

- Clinically indicated testing (e.g., depakote, lithium, or tegretol level, liver function tests, EKG, metabolic monitoring)
- Completing Abnormal Involuntary Movement Scale (AIMS) when indicated

Teleclinician Satisfaction

Teleclinician satisfaction and well-being have received some attention, but more research is needed to better understand factors that contribute to teleclinician satisfaction, engagement, and burnout [9]. For example, TBH can enhance the teleclinician's job satisfaction and well-being by eliminating the need to commute and improving scheduling flexibility [10]. However, teleclinicians can also experience professional and social isolation, and a blurring of the distinction between occupational and personal spaces [9]. Isolation can lead to dissatisfaction with delivering care remotely, which may also be exacerbated by other program factors such as relationship dynamics with staff of the facility-based OS, or challenges with ICT. Accordingly, an important aspect of M & E for TBH is to assess teleclinician satisfaction, engagement, and well-being. As with patient satisfaction, a combination of quantitative and qualitative measures is can be used, depending on the objectives and goals of data collection.

Information and Communication Technologies

ICT monitoring is essential to evaluate the software for security, ensure hardware maintenance, and maintain the quality of connectivity (see Toolbox 8.1). Monitoring helps anticipate potential needs for technological support and guides training requirements on ICT updates [4]. In addition, surveying all users, including patients, OS staff, and teleclinicians, can help optimize user experience and improve satisfaction with ICT.

Toolbox 8.1 ICT Quality Checklist
- Provide training for staff at onboarding and annually on HIPAA, HITECH, and data privacy.
- Monitor adherence to electronic data security and hardware security.
- Monitor and update firewall, antivirus software, and security patches.
- Monitor Internet connectivity and security.
- Maintain and regularly update hardware.
- Ensure that videoconferencing, patient portals, telephone, and text-based software are secure and HIPAA/HITECH compliant.
- Monitor the type, frequency, and resolution associated with technical issues reported by users.
- Monitor response times for IT support.
- Survey and optimize user experience for patients, OS staff, and teleclinicians.

For facility-based services, the information technology (IT) team or a dedicated team member should ensure that ICT components are monitored regularly, both at the OS and teleclinician sides. For home-based services, the teleclinician should ensure that they monitor ICT components with regard to their own technology and should inform patients of both the ICT requirements needed to conduct sessions effectively and securely, as well as of the potential risks associated with digital communication.

Security

Ensure that all those involved in the delivery of TBH are regularly trained on HIPAA, HITECH, and data privacy. This should include training during onboarding, prior to any PHI handling. In addition, conduct a mandatory annual training on these issues for all team members and incorporate test cases and examples in the training. Should testing reveal any gaps in knowledge, these should be addressed immediately and additional training should be offered.

Ensure that OS staff and teleclinicians are trained on cybersecurity. All staff working with technology should monitor their electronic communications for potentially harmful content, such as phishing, and for any security breach, and should report any suspicious activity to the IT department, compliance officer, or other designated staff member. For home-based services, the teleclinician should document any instances wherein either they or their patient detects suspicious or unusual communication. The teleclinician should use such instances as a prompt to run cybersecurity checks on their ICT and urge their patient to do the same.

Under HIPAA, certain security incidents or breaches may require specific reporting and mitigation steps [11]. Further discussion of security measures and monitoring for software and hardware can be found in Chap. 6.

Support

Facility-based TBH programs generally include technological support. This support may range from a single IT team member to a call center with multiple levels of support. Regardless of the degree of IT support available to an organization, we recommend a system of documenting the type, frequency, response time, and resolution of IT issues. Tracking these data points provides insights into potential trends in accessing and using the technology. It may be used to inform decisions on the ICT used to deliver TBH services, including choice of hardware and software, connectivity options, necessary updates or upgrades, and additional staff and teleclinician training.

Cultural and Regulatory Framework

As explained in Chap. 7, cultural appropriateness of TBH is instrumental in providing BHS that improve access, utilization, and satisfaction of patients from culturally and linguistically diverse communities (see Toolbox 8.2).

> **Toolbox 8.2 Outcome Measures Examined Through a Cultural Lens [12]**
> - Patient satisfaction
> - Clinician satisfaction
> - Care process, such as care coordination, treatment adherence, and no-shows
> - Communication, such as rapport
> - Symptom tracking
> - Cost, such as ICT costs
> - Administrative factors, such as staffing and facility management

Cultural Framework

Demographic changes in the United States will continue to challenge healthcare systems to not only incorporate culturally competent services, such as language services and culturally appropriate clinicians but also to regularly evaluate these services, including staffing needs and care interventions [12]. The outcome measures to evaluate TBH programs that are discussed throughout this chapter can be examined through a cultural perspective. This applies to patient satisfaction, patient engagement, teleclinician satisfaction, symptom tracking, and costs.

For quality assurance of culturally appropriate BHS, ensure that OS staff and teleclinician receive sufficient training on culturally appropriate care. It is worth acknowledging that historically such training courses have varied in scope and quality, with some erroneously assuming or suggesting that members of major ethnic and racial groups uniformly share the same characteristics. This is problematic, as in reality, most people incorporate multiple social identities, individual histories, and backgrounds that shape their attitudes, beliefs, and values in ways that may not always align with the group or community they belong to [13, 14]. As such, maintaining a curious, open, and humble attitude is instrumental for the provision of effective BHS.

Ensure the availability of well-trained interpreters and cultural facilitators, when needed. Avoid using "informal" interpreters, such as family members, nurses, or any personnel without sufficient training, as they would run the risk of miscommunicating the complaints, de-emphasizing information or missing culture-specific metaphors [12]. Utilize screening tools that are validated in appropriate linguistic and cultural settings. For example, the PHQ-9 is available in many languages and its use has demonstrated its validity across different linguistic and cultural settings [15, 16].

Regulatory Compliance

The telehealth regulatory landscape continues to evolve, particularly since the start of the COVID-19 pandemic. OS support staff, including compliance and credentialing team members, and teleclinicians should ensure they are following the most current jurisdiction-specific and federal regulations dictating the practice of

TBH. Attention should also be paid to evolving guidelines and reimbursement changes from commercial and public payers, and to guidance issued by professional societies and jurisdiction-specific professional boards. Monitoring these guidelines and regulations not only ensures TBH program compliance but may also provide up-to-date resources and support for your TBH program.

Teleclinician Considerations

Considerations for monitoring and quality assurance of a teleclinician's performance are addressed earlier in this chapter; however, of equal importance is vetting the teleclinician prior to deploying your TBH program through different processes, including but not limited to background checks, reference checks, personal disclosures, malpractice history, and National Practitioner Data Bank reports. Initial verification of teleclinician credentials should be followed by regular monitoring of such credentials. This may include the maintenance of appropriate licensure, obtaining required continuing education credits, and maintaining necessary board certification or other credentials. Other examples include tracking the completion and annual review of collaborative agreements, if the teleclinician is participating in a collaborative relationship, the maintenance of facility privileges and payer credentials, and continuous monitoring for any adverse actions associated with the clinician, such as regular Office of Inspector General reporting. Generally, the monitoring of these items falls within an organization's Credentialing Department or Medical Affairs Department, which collects and maintains documentation on the clinician's credentials. Organizations may find it beneficial to use comprehensive software solutions to facilitate these tasks. While the administrative support and software required to verify and monitor clinician credentials may require some financial investment, the ability of these solutions to cross-reference multiple sources may ultimately save organizations time and enable more rapid scaling of TBH programs. However an organization chooses to complete the processes of verifying and monitoring teleclinician credentials, remember that these quality assurance processes are vital in ensuring a clinician is and remains qualified to deliver care.

Other Considerations

Similar to in-person care, consider regular training on compliance and ethics for all staff who may come in contact with patients and PHI. While such training has its own quality assurance merits, it may also be required for some organizations that contract with Medicare or as part of other regulatory compliance (see Toolbox 8.3) [17]. For example, CMS has specific requirements for a compliance program for certain organizations, including training on code of conduct, conflict of interest, and waste, fraud, and abuse [18, 19]. Remember that some states and payers may have further regulatory and training requirements.

> **Toolbox 8.3 Regulatory Quality Checklist**
> - Ensure licensure requirements are met
> - Ensure collaborative agreements are completed and signed
> - Ensure teleclinician is privileged with the facility and credentialed with payers
> - Ensure training on HIPAA, security, privacy, HITECH
> - Monitor compliance with federal HIPAA and HITECH requirements
> - Monitor compliance with state or other jurisdiction privacy laws
> - Ensure adherence to HHS, Medicare, Medicaid, and private payer guidelines
> - Ensure compliance with federal and jurisdiction-specific prescribing guidelines

References

1. Haidous M, Tawil M, Naal H, Mahmoud H. A review of evaluation approaches for telemental health programs. Int J Psychiat Clin Pract. 2021;25:195–205.
2. Mahmoud H, Vogt EL, Dahdouh R, Raymond ML. Using continuous quality improvement to design and implement a telepsychiatry program in rural Illinois. Psychiatr Serv. 2020;appi.ps.2019002.

3. Mahmoud H, Naal H, Cerda S. Planning and implementing telepsychiatry in a community mental health setting. a case study report. Community Mental Health J [Internet]. 2020;(0123456789). https://doi.org/10.1007/s10597-020-00709-1

4. Mahmoud H, Whaibeh E, Mitchel B. Ensuring successful telepsychiatry program implementation: critical components and considerations. Curr Treatment Opt Psychiat. 2020;

5. Fortney JC, Pyne JM, Turner EE, Farris KM, Normoyle TM, Avery MD, et al. Telepsychiatry integration of mental health services into rural primary care settings. Int Rev Psychiatry. 2015;27(6):525–39.

6. Mahmoud H, Vogt E. Telepsychiatry: an innovative approach to addressing the opioid crisis. J Behav Health Serv Res. 2019;46(4):680–5.

7. O'Reilly R, Bishop J, Maddox K, Hutchinson L, Fisman M, Takhar J. Is telepsychiatry equivalent to face-to-face psychiatry? Results from a randomized controlled equivalence trial. Psychiatr Serv. 2007;58(6):836–43.

8. Hilty DM, Ferrer DC, Parish MB, Johnston B, Callahan EJ, Yellowlees PM. The effectiveness of telemental health: a 2013 review. Telemedicine and e-Health. 2013;19(6):444–54.

9. Vogt EL, Mahmoud H, Elhaj O. Telepsychiatry: implications for psychiatrist burnout and well-being. Psychiatr Serv. 2019;70(5):422–4.

10. Mahmoud H, Naal H, Mitchel B. Evaluating a multicomponent strategy to address burnout, job engagement, and job satisfaction among telepsychiatrists. J Psychiatr Pract. 2021.

11. HHS. HITECH Act Enforcement Interim Final Rule. U.S Department of Health & Human Services. 2017.

12. Hilty DM, Gentry MT, McKean AJ, Cowan KE, Lim RF, Lu FG. Telehealth for rural diverse populations: telebehavioral and cultural competencies, clinical outcomes and administrative approaches. mHealth. 2020;6.

13. Annamalai A, Terasaki G. Culturally appropriate care. In: Refugee health care. Cham: Springer International Publishing; 2020.

14. Mendoza NS, Moreno FA, Hishaw GA, Gaw AC, Fortuna LR, Skubel A, et al. Affirmative care across cultures: broadening application. Focus. 2020;18(1).

15. Wulsin L, Somoza E, Heck J. The feasibility of using the Spanish PHQ-9 to screen for depression in primary care in Honduras. The primary care companion to. J Clin Psychiatry. 2002;04(05).

16. Arthurs E, Steele RJ, Hudson M, Baron M, Thombs BD. Are scores on English and French versions of the PHQ-9 comparable? An assessment of differential item functioning. PLoS One. 2012;7(12).

17. Dowell M. Federally qualified Health center and Rural Health center Telemedicine compliance and legal issues. J Healthcare Complianc. 2019.

18. CMS. Medicare fraud & abuse: prevent, detect, report. 2021.

19. CMS. Medicare Parts C and D General Compliance Training Web-Based Training Course. 2019.

Current Trends and Anticipated Directions in TBH

9

Hossam Mahmoud

Current Trends

The exponential increase in the adoption and utilization of TBH that accompanied the COVID-19 pandemic is likely to irreversibly place ICT at the heart of BHS delivery. Since March 2020, the conversation about TBH has shifted from whether BHS can be delivered remotely in a manner that is feasible and that maintains quality of care, to *how* TBH can be best implemented to optimize integration, efficiency, cost-effectiveness, and quality of care. In addition to the increased adoption of more "traditional" TBH, in the form of direct patient care through synchronous videoconferencing, there is also wider appreciation for the value of TBH in delivering care and support across the BH continuum, from pre-clinical symptoms to severe conditions, using different care models and population health approaches.

Care Management

ICT inherent to the delivery of TBH are being used to monitor and improve the quality of care, through data tracking and predictive analytics. We have seen an expansion in the use of virtual care

H. Mahmoud (✉)
Tufts University School of Medicine, Boston, MA, USA

© The Author(s), under exclusive license to Springer Nature Switzerland AG 2022
H. Mahmoud et al. (eds.), *Essentials of Telebehavioral Health*,
https://doi.org/10.1007/978-3-030-97325-4_9

management that utilizes analytic and predictive data to proactively identify and stratify patients, depending on acuity of symptoms and anticipated patient needs, with the premise that early identification and intervention can lead to better healthcare outcomes and decreased costs. While readers may disagree on whether, strictly speaking, virtual care management falls under TBH, such virtual programs can support care delivery and allow for more targeted care by providing education, patient engagement, and care navigation services, in order to triage patients to the BHS, including TBH services, that are appropriate for them.

Digital Health Solutions

There has been an increase in the number of digital solutions that offer self-navigated management and tracking tools to address milder BH symptoms and conditions and to support emotional health and well-being. These self-navigated solutions can tackle stress, resilience building, mild depressive and anxiety symptoms, and insomnia, to name a few [1–3]. Depending on the digital health solution, the tools can range from psychoeducational videos, guided meditation, and self-help-type modules to more formal modules using cognitive behavioral therapy, motivational interviewing, and mindfulness approaches. The advantages of such tools include the fact that they are convenient and are available on demand 24/7 through phones, tablets, and computers. They do not require making appointments and bypass the stigma associated with seeking BHS.

Because consistent engagement with these digital solutions can be an issue, some solutions have also incorporated into their delivery models the use of non-licensed telecoaches, to increase engagement with self-navigated modules and provide navigation and support services. However, it is important to point out that the use of non-clinicians, such as telecoaches, peer support specialists and care navigators to enhance treatment engagement and support, has been expanding across TBH services, including those delivered by teleclinicians via videoconferencing. These non-clinicians may provide additional support between appointments and may also assist with care coordination, care navigation, inter-appointment questions, BH resources and educational material, and triage.

Asynchronous Care

We have seen an increase in the acceptability and utilization of non-appointment-based asynchronous TBH services for the delivery of direct patient care. Asynchronous care uses store and forward ICT in the form of video messages, audio messages, emailing, and other messaging services. The advantage of such asynchronous communication modalities is that they eliminate the scheduling "friction" that may occur when trying to set up a live session with a teleclinician, thus increasing the convenience of receiving care. While some patients prefer treatment delivered synchronously, the availability of asynchronous care offers patients additional treatment choices with increased convenience. Asynchronous care is increasingly being used to deliver psychotherapy services, such as cognitive-behavioral therapy. In addition, hybrid models of synchronous and asynchronous care delivery are increasingly being used for psychiatric medication management.

Higher Levels of Care

With the COVID-19 pandemic, there has been a significant increase in the utilization and acceptance of TBH at more intensive levels of care, such as IOPs and PHPs [4], as well as residential facilities and inpatient psychiatric units. Studies suggest positive outcomes at higher levels of care, with symptom reduction and patient satisfaction [5]. With such levels of care, we might encounter cases whereby the OS may change during treatment, especially with hybrid TBH and in-person programs. For example, psychotherapy services can be delivered at a PHP-level intensity while the patient is at home (home-based services); alternatively, while the patient is at a PHP facility (facility-based services), a particular teleclinician might deliver psychotherapy from a remote location.

Since programming higher levels of care, such as IOP and PHP, usually includes family and group psychotherapy, the expanded TBH implementation at these levels of care that occurred during the COVID-19 pandemic is likely to provide more data not only on TBH implementation at higher levels of care but also on TBH utility in group settings. This will have further implications on TBH application moving forward as there has been an increased interest in employing TBH for family and couple psychotherapy [6].

Tele-MAT

We have noted an increase in the use of TBH to deliver treatment for SUD, including MAT for OUD. This is likely due to a confluence of factors, including care delivery disruptions during the COVID-19 pandemic, increased rates of SUD, persistent stigma-related barriers, and shortage of addiction specialists, especially buprenorphine-waivered prescribers. Regulatory and reimbursement changes during the pandemic have supported this expansion by enhancing reimbursement for TBH services, lifting the restrictions on OS types and locations, and suspending the limitations on prescribing controlled substances—including buprenorphine—set by the Ryan Haight Act [7, 8]. Furthermore, in April 2021, HHS issued guidance adjusting the DEA waiver requirement for prescribing buprenorphine for the treatment of OUD in order to increase access to MAT. This guidance will likely further facilitate buprenorphine prescribing through TBH.

Consultative Models

We have noted an increased recognition of the value of utilizing TBH to deliver consultation services, including through asynchronous e-consults, synchronous and asynchronous video-based curbside consults, and the collaborative care model (CoCM). With e-consults the psychiatric teleclinician typically provides support in an asynchronous manner using the EHR, after reviewing the consult questions and conducting a chart review. Video-based curbside consults can be delivered both synchronously and asynchronously, depending on the preference of the clinicians, the urgency of the consult and the availability of the psychiatric tele-clinician. The CoCM has expanded and standardized the delivery of consultative BH services into primary care settings, with the addition of BH care managers imbedded within primary care settings and the incorporation of standardized tools to track clinical outcomes. These trends are in line with the need to meet patients' BH needs in the context of the shortage of BH clinicians, and they reflect a move toward increased cross-specialty care integration and outcomes-based care [9].

Value-Based Care

There has been an increased interest among payers and some healthcare systems in value-based programs that emphasize the quality of care provided rather than the volume of patients served or numbers of sessions conducted. Sometimes referred to as outcomes-based arrangements, such programs provide payments to incentivize the quality of care delivered, as opposed to fee-for-service arrangements. While the interest in value-based care is by no means restricted to TBH, remote service delivery may be the catalyst to facilitate the expansion of outcomes-based payment models. TBH is seen as an opportunity to capitalize on the use of ICT inherent to the delivery of remote services to monitor both process and outcome data and to incorporate data analytics into TBH program design, facilitating the tracking of the quality and cost of care.

Future Directions

At the time of writing this book, TBH continues to be widely utilized, and we anticipate a continued increase in the use of ICT to deliver a variety of BHS to meet patient needs. Even after the COVID-19 pandemic is contained, TBH utilization is unlikely to return to pre-pandemic levels, particularly after the perceived utility and perceived ease of use of TBH have been solidly established, and the "forced" adoption has increased TBH acceptability among patients, clinicians, facilities, and payers. Future directions in TBH and healthcare innovations will likely be guided by future regulatory, reimbursement, and sociocultural factors. Other factors include innovations in ICT, investment in healthcare, technology availability, and access to broadband Internet connectivity.

The regulatory landscape shaping the delivery of TBH services continues to evolve and appears to be developing in a manner that supports further expansion of TBH. There appears to be wider recognition that future TBH-related laws and regulations need to be evidence-based, building on lessons learned from the pandemic-related regulatory measures and incorporating evidence from research on the impact of such measures on access to care, as well as on the quality and cost of care. Investment in healthcare technologies and innovations increased to record levels during the COVID-19 pandemic, and this growth is expected to continue at least in the near future. And while there have been many success stories demonstrating TBH as decreasing some healthcare disparities, there is an increased recognition that the expansion and reliance on TBH have created new healthcare disparities. These are referred to as the "digital divide" that results when different patients or patient populations have varying degrees of proficiency in ICT use or varying access to ICT and Internet connectivity from safe secure spaces. In turn, this leaves some patient populations with ongoing access issues, including patients from lower socioeconomic backgrounds, geriatric populations, rural communities, and ethnic and racial minorities. For example, LGBTQ youth may face difficulties accessing TBH services as some homes where LGBTQ individuals reside may not constitute private safe spaces from which to access care. We also recognize the risk that cultural and linguistic minorities may continue to be on the underserved side of that digital divide. In recognition of this divide, and in an attempt to mitigate it, there has been an increased interest in "audio-only telehealth," which has been reimbursed during the COVID-19 pandemic, with some support for continued coverage for audio-only sessions even after the resolution of the public health emergency [10–12].

Moving forward, we anticipated a trend toward hybridization of care delivery, such as hybrid in-person and TBH care, hybrid synchronous and asynchronous care, and hybrid virtual direct care and consultative models. In fact, the APA expects the typical psychiatric practice after the COVID-19 pandemic to deliver a hybrid model that incorporates in-person, video, and telephone visits [13]. In addition, while TBH will continue to be used by teleclinicians and healthcare facilities to expand access to care, and by payers to meet network adequacy requirements, reimbursement structures are likely to follow the healthcare industry trend away from fee-for-service and toward measurement-based care and value-based arrangements.

Remote monitoring is an expanding area of telehealth. Remote monitoring, or tele-supervision, involves the continuous evaluation of a patient's clinical status using either objective or subjective data points collected from the patient's remote location and securely transmitted to the evaluating clinician. Remote monitoring has been particularly useful for patients living in rural or under-resourced areas, where it may be difficult to access adequately trained clinicians for follow-up, and for patients with chronic conditions who wish to remain in the comfort of their homes rather than the hospital [14]. While remote monitoring for BHS has not been widely implemented, there is increasing interest in "digital phenotyping" in BH [15]. An example is using smartphones to collect objective data on mood, behavior, and cognition. Phone sensors can track levels of activity and location; voice and speech analysis provides data on coherence, sentiment, and prosody; and human–computer interaction offers data on attention, memory, and reaction times [15]. Such interactions would track subtle changes in scrolling and typing as proxy indicators of affective states and cognitive traits [15]. While more research is needed to understand the utility and limitations of digital phenotyping, it is anticipated that investment in such solutions is going to expand due to expectations of cost-efficiency and scalability of phone-based phenotyping [16].

Another anticipated trend is an increase in the application of artificial intelligence (AI) and machine learning, which has been generating interest for the past decade [17]. The applications have been relatively focused on some digital health components, text-enabled services, and behavioral analysis and modeling for treatment interventions [18] to create a more individualized patient experience and support some aspects of TBH service delivery. Some applications remain relatively limited at the time of writing this book as scalability continues to be constrained by costs, feasibility, and the need for further research and guidelines on the use of AI [15]. However, the near future is likely to bring expanded application of AI and machine learning to support quality, efficiency, and experience of TBH service delivery. This is likely to be accompanied with an increase in the use of analytic and predictive data to support planning, implementation, monitoring, and continuous refining of TBH programs.

The past few years have certainly witnessed a transformation in BH. We have seen ICT becoming integral to BHS, shifting the manner in which BHS are delivered and opening the door for further innovations in care delivery aimed at improving care and decreasing costs. Regardless of the service, approach, or technology utilized, we hope that the future directions of TBH continue to honor the historical purpose of TBH: to serve as a tool to expand access to BHS, improve ease of accessing care, bypass stigma, and decrease healthcare disparities.

References

1. Duffy D, Enrique A, Connell S, Connolly C, Richards D. Internet-delivered cognitive behavior therapy as a prequel to face-to-face therapy for depression and anxiety: a naturalistic observation. Front Psych. 2020;10.
2. Eilert N, Enrique A, Wogan R, Mooney O, Timulak L, Richards D. The effectiveness of Internet-delivered treatment for generalized anxiety disorder: an updated systematic review and meta-analysis. Depress Anxiety. 2021;38(2).
3. Enrique A, Mooney O, Salamanca-Sanabria A, Lee CT, Farrell S, Richards D. Assessing the efficacy and acceptability of an internet-delivered intervention for resilience among college students: a pilot randomised control trial protocol. Internet Interv. 2019;17.

4. Hom MA, Weiss RB, Millman ZB, Christensen K, Lewis EJ, Cho S, et al. Development of a virtual partial hospital program for an acute psychiatric population: Lessons learned and future directions for telepsychotherapy. J Psychother Integration. 2020;30(2).

5. Zimmerman M, Terrill D, D'avanzato C, Tirpak J. Telehealth treatment of patients in an intensive acute care psychiatric setting during the COVID-19 pandemic: comparative safety and effectiveness to in-person treatment. J Clin Psychiatry. 2021.

6. Hertlein KM, Drude KP, Hilty DM, Maheu MM. Toward proficiency in telebehavioral health: applying interprofessional competencies in couple and family therapy. J Marital Fam Ther. 2021;47(2).

7. Mahmoud H, Vogt E. Telepsychiatry: an innovative approach to addressing the opioid crisis. J Behav Health Serv Res. 2019;46(4):680–5.

8. Whaibeh E, Mahmoud H, Naal H. Telemental health in the context of a pandemic: the COVID-19 experience. Curr Treatment Opt Psychiat. 2020;7(2):198–202.

9. Mahmoud H, Vogt EL, Dahdouh R, Raymond ML. Using continuous quality improvement to design and implement a telepsychiatry program in rural Illinois. Psychiatr Serv. 2020;71(8):860–3.

10. Robeznieks A. Why audio-only telehealth visits must continue. American Medical Association.

11. Wicklund E. AMA lobbies CMS to extend medicare coverage for audio-only telehealth. mHealth Intelligence; 2021.

12. AHIP. Using telehealth to deliver affordable, high-quality care. America's Health Insurance Plans; 2021.

13. Moran M. Vaccinating patients with SMI: one public hospital's experience. Psychiatr News. 2021;56(5).

14. Augusterfer EF, O'Neal CR, Martin SW, Sheikh TL, Mollica RF. The role of telemental health, tele-consultation, and Tele-supervision in post-disaster and low-resource settings. Curr Psychiat Rep. 2020;22.

15. Insel TR. Digital phenotyping: technology for a new science of behavior. JAMA. 2017;318:1215–6.

16. Onnela J-P, Rauch SL. Harnessing smartphone-based digital phenotyping to enhance behavioral and mental health. Neuropsychopharmacology. 2016;41(7).

17. Luxton DD, Skopp NA, Maguen S. Gender differences in depression and PTSD symptoms following combat exposure. Depress Anxiety. 2010;27(11):1027–33.

18. Malgaroli M, Hull TD, Schultebraucks K. Digital health and artificial intelligence for PTSD: improving treatment delivery through personalization. Psychiatr Ann. 2021;51(1).

Appendix

Index and Resources

Chapter 2: Telebehavioral Health: The Basics

A timeline of the steps taken by the Federal government to support telehealth during the COVID-19 pandemic

https://www.beckershospitalreview.com/telehealth/a-timeline-of-telehealth-support-from-the-federal-government-during-the-pandemic.html

Chapter 3: The Originating site

Database of EHR softwares:

https://surescripts.com/network-alliance/eprescribing-prescriber-software

APA guidance on the components of clinical documentation in TBH:

https://www.psychiatry.org/psychiatrists/practice/telepsychiatry/toolkit/clinical-documentation

EPCS information:

https://www.deadiversion.usdoj.gov/ecomm/e_rx/thirdparty.htm

Database of e-prescribing softwares:

https://surescripts.com/network-alliance/eprescribing-prescriber-software

Chapter 5: The Teleclincian

Examples of HHS Model Notices of Privacy Practices: https://www.hhs.gov/hipaa/for-professionals/privacy/guidance/model-notices-privacy-practices/index.html

The American Academy of Child and Adolescent Psychiatry provides resources and templates on consent for treatment, patient information, ROI, and other practice management templates: https://www.aacap.org/aacap/Clinical_Practice_Center/Business_of_Practice/Practice_Forms_HIPAA_Disclosures.aspx

Testing Internet Speed

https://beta.speedtest.net/

Resources for identifying and contacting local emergency services

www.usacops.com

www.policelocator.com

Database of e-prescribing softwares:

https://surescripts.com/network-alliance/eprescribing-prescriber-software

APA guidance on the components of clinical documentation in TBH:

https://www.psychiatry.org/psychiatrists/practice/telepsychiatry/toolkit/clinical-documentation

Database of EHR softwares: https://surescripts.com/network-alliance/eprescribing-prescriber-software

Billing Resources

- The Centers for Medicare & Medicaid Services https://www.cms.gov/Medicare/Medicare-General-Information/Telehealth
- American Psychiatric Association https://www.psychiatry.org/psychiatrists/practice/telepsychiatry/blog/apa-resources-on-telepsychiatry-and-covid-19
- American Psychological Association https://www.apa.org/monitor/2020/06/covid-telepsychology
- Center for Connected Health Policy https://www.cchpca.org/ Resources on Well-being and Burnout

- American Psychiatric Association https://www.psychiatry.org/psychiatrists/practice/well-being-and-burnout

- The National Academy of Medicine https://nam.edu/systems-approaches-to-improve-patient-care-by-supporting-clinician-well-being/
- American Medical Association https://www.ama-assn.org/practice-management/physician-health/6-big-things-must-change-beat-physician-burnout

Chapter 6: Information and Communications Technologies

Planning and Implementing Telepsychiatry in a Community Mental Health Setting: A Case Study Report https://pubmed.ncbi.nlm.nih.gov/32897476/

Examples of HIPAA-compliant platforms:

https://www.camft.org/Resources/Legal-Articles/Telehealth-HIPAA-and-Compliant-Telehealth-Platforms

Testing Internet Speed

www.speedtest.net

Cybersecurity Checklist

https://www.healthit.gov/sites/default/files/basic-security-for-the-small-healthcare-practice-checklists.pdf

CMS Rules on Security, Privacy and Breach Notification https://www.cms.gov/outreach-and-education/medicare-learning-network-mln/mlnproducts/downloads/hipaaprivacyand-securitytextonly.pdf

Chapter 7: Cultural and Regulatory Frameworks

The Interstate Medical Licensure Compact

https://www.imlcc.org/a-faster-pathway-to-physician-licensure/

State by state Information on collaboration and supervision requirements for nurse practitioners

https://www.aanp.org/advocacy/state/state-practice-environment

Resources on culturally affirming care

- American Psychiatric Association. Best Practice Highlights for Treating Diverse Patient Populations https://www.psychiatry.org/psychiatrists/cultural-competency/education/best-practice-highlights

- American Psychiatric Association. Cultural Formulation Interview. (2013). http://www.multiculturalmentalhealth.ca/wp-content/uploads/2013/10/2013_DSM5_CFI_InformantVersion.pdf.
- American Psychiatric Association. Cultural Formulation Interview Supplementary Modules 2013. http://www.multiculturalmentalhealth.ca/wp-content/uploads/2013/10/2013_CFI_supplementarymodules.pdf.
- National Association of Social Workers. Standards and Indicators of Cultural Competence in Social Work Practice 2015 https://www.socialworkers.org/LinkClick.aspx?fileticket=PonPTDEBrn4%3D&portalid=0
- American Psychological Association. Guidelines for Providers of Psychological Services to Ethnic, Linguistic, and Culturally Diverse Populations 2017. http://www.apa.org/pi/oema/resources/policy/provider-guidelines.aspx.
- American Counseling Association. Code of Ethics 2014. https://www.counseling.org/resources/aca-code-of-ethics.pdf.

Chapter 8: Monitoring and Evaluation and Quality Assurance

Resources on clinical, professional, regulatory and reimbursement guidelines for TBH

- American Psychiatric Association:
  - Telepsychiatry Toolkit
    https://www.psychiatry.org/psychiatrists/practice/telepsychiatry/toolkit
  - Telemental Health Guide
    https://www.psychiatry.org/psychiatrists/practice/telepsychiatry/blog/apa-and-ata-release-new-telemental-health-guide
- American Telemedicine Association
  - ATA practice guidelines for video-based online mental health services
    https://pubmed.ncbi.nlm.nih.gov/32897476/

- Centers for Medicare and Medicaid Services
  - Medicare Telemedicine Health Care Provider Fact Sheet
    https://www.cms.gov/newsroom/fact-sheets/medicare-telemedicine-health-care-provider-fact-sheet
  - Quality Measures: Traditional MIPS Requirements
    https://qpp.cms.gov/mips/quality-requirements

Planning and Implementing Telepsychiatry in a Community Mental Health Setting: A Case Study Report https://pubmed.ncbi.nlm.nih.gov/32897476/.

Using Continuous Quality Improvement to Design and Implement a Telepsychiatry Program in Rural Illinois https://ps.psychiatryonline.org/doi/10.1176/appi.ps.201900231.

Glossary

Asynchronous services The delivery of services in a "store-and-forward" manner.

Collaborative care model A measurement-based integrated care model, from the University of Washington, that is based on the collaboration of a triad made of a primary care provider, embedded behavioral health specialist and a psychiatric consultant, using a patient registry.

COVID-19 The 2019 novel coronavirus disease, declared a pandemic by the World Health Organization on February 11, 2020.

Distant site The physical location, from which the teleclinician is delivering TBH services.

E-consult Asynchronous consultation between healthcare professionals, typically completed via electronic health record.

HIPAA The Health Insurance Portability and Accountability Act, a Federal law that regulates the protection, storage and communication of patient health information.

HITECH The Health Information Technology for Economic and Clinical Health Act, a Federal law aimed at promoting the adoption and use of health information technology, with an emphasis on the privacy and security of health information transmitted by electronic means.

Home-based TBH TBH services delivered to an originating site that is not a healthcare facility. This definition has been used to include patient homes, offices or other private locations outside a healthcare facility. Synonym: TBH in clinically unsupervised settings.

© The Editor(s) (if applicable) and The Author(s), under exclusive license to Springer Nature Switzerland AG 2022
H. Mahmoud et al. (eds.), *Essentials of Telebehavioral Health*,
https://doi.org/10.1007/978-3-030-97325-4

The Interstate Medical Licensure Compact A streamlined and expedited pathway to physician licensing based on an agreement among multiple United States and territories.

Medication-assisted treatment The use of medications alongside psychotherapy for treating opioid use disorders. A more expanded definition includes medications used for the treatment of substance use disorders more broadly. Examples include disulfiram, acamprosate, and naltrexone for alcohol use disorder; methadone, buprenorphine, and naltrexone for opioid use disorder; and naloxone opioid overdose prevention.

Originating site The physical or "brick-and-mortar" location where patients are located at the time of receiving TBH services

Patient support person A friend, family, or community member identified by the patient. A PSP who can assist in emergencies. The PSP can provide assistance in assessing the emergency or possibly initiating emergency service calls from the patient's location.

Protected health information Individually identifiable data pertaining to the health status of a person that a HIPAA-covered entity collects, creates, maintains, or transmits, in the context of healthcare service delivery, payment, or operations.

The Ryan Haight Online Pharmacy Consumer Protection Act of 2008 A federal law that—with some exceptions—prohibits prescribers from prescribing controlled substances without first conducting an in-person evaluation. unless the circumstance meets one of the 7 exceptions (Levine & Wein 2020)

Synchronous services Services delivered in real time.

Telebehavioral health The use of information and communications technologies, including but not limited to, videoconferencing in order to deliver behavioral health services remotely. Other terms used under the umbrella of TBH also include electronic health (e-health), mobile health (m-health), and digital health. Synonyms: telepsychiatry, telemental health, or virtual behavioral health.

Value-based care or value-based program A program in which
payments incentivize the quality of care delivered. Value-based
arrangements are also referred to as outcomes-based arrangements, and are at times contrasted with fee-for-services
arrangements.

Index